Working with
Adults with
Asperger Syndrome

Working with Adults with Asperger Syndrome

A PRACTICAL TOOLKIT

▶ Carol Hagland

▶ Zillah Webb

Jessica Kingsley Publishers
London and Philadelphia

First published in 2009
by Jessica Kingsley Publishers
116 Pentonville Road
London N1 9JB, UK
and
400 Market Street, Suite 400
Philadelphia, PA 19106, USA

www.jkp.com

Library of Congress Cataloging in Publication Data
Hagland, Carol.
  Working with adults with Asperger syndrome : a practical toolkit / Carol Hagland and Zillah Webb.
    p. cm.
  Includes bibliographical references and index.
  ISBN 978-1-84905-036-4 (pb : alk. paper) 1. Asperger's syndrome--Popular works. I. Webb, Zillah. II. Title.
  RC553.A88H356 2009
  616.85'8832--dc22

                                                        2009007243

British Library Cataloguing in Publication Data
A CIP catalogue record for this book is available from the British Library

ISBN 978 1 84905 036 4

Printed and bound in Great Britain by
Athenaeum Press, Gateshead, Tyne and Wear

Acknowledgements

With special acknowledgements to Surrey and Borders Partnership NHS Trust who kindly supported the development of much of this workbook.

This workbook was developed from an idea originally proposed by Dr Vicky Tozer. The authors would also like to acknowledge the substantial contribution of Nicole Krokidis who assisted in gathering information and compiling the first draft of the workbook.

Thanks are due in addition to Thomas Moore, of Surrey Social Services, for facilitating the pilot group through his 'Autism Champions' network. The contributions of the members of the pilot 'Asperger's Champions' group were invaluable in finding which exercises worked and where the text needed clarification or elaboration.

Finally we gratefully acknowledge the contribution of all the individuals with Asperger syndrome who we have worked with, and the people who support them.

Contents

Confidentiality Statement

In order to illustrate some of the problems experienced by people with Asperger syndrome and the people who care for them we have included case examples throughout this guide.

While these examples are drawn from the experiences of real people with Asperger syndrome, they have been altered. All names are fictitious and details have been changed to maintain confidentiality and anonymity of individuals and organisations. Most examples are composites of different people's experiences.

Introduction

WHAT IS ASPERGER SYNDROME?

Asperger syndrome (AS) is not a mental illness. It is a developmental disorder. That means that people are born with it. It is the result of differences in the way that the brain works, which affect the way they learn about, and interact with the world around them. The causes are not known for sure. Sometimes the condition seems to develop after a difficult birth, but it does seem to run in some families, so may have a genetic component too.

People with AS show a number of typical behavioural characteristics. There is no universally agreed way of identifying AS, but a useful set of criteria were developed by Gillberg and Gillberg (1986). These criteria can be used to aid diagnosis, and it is recommended that anyone interested in diagnosis should read their original work.

Gillberg and Gillberg described a pattern of difficulties that people with AS usually have. These include a range of social problems, such as appearing self-centred or selfish, and having difficulty in interacting with other people. Largely these difficulties arise because the person with AS does not pick up the social signals that others give. They sometimes behave in ways that seem inappropriate and may not always want to make a lot of friends, being happy with their own company.

People with AS usually have a special interest that occupies their time and thoughts a great deal. They may neglect other activities because of their obsession with this topic, and often learn many facts off by heart. Given the chance they will talk at length about this topic, often driving other people away as a result.

Routine and repetition are also characteristic of those with AS, and they will often have a set pattern of activities during the day that they like to follow. They may become upset if this routine has to change, and may try and insist that others follow their routines too.

Language development usually seems fairly normal in people with AS, but sometimes it can be delayed, and although they develop superficially good expressive speech, the content of their speech can be unusual, and may sound odd. Often the person sounds rather formal, and may speak rather loudly and monotonously. Most people with AS have some problems with the understanding of language, however, especially if sentences are long or complicated.

HOW SHOULD THIS BOOK BE USED?

The major aim of this workbook is to assist those who support people with AS to have a better understanding of the condition and of their client's needs.

People with AS can be extremely intelligent and talented. Even those who are not can seem more able than they are. They often talk fluently and know a lot about their chosen interests. As a result it is easy to overestimate an AS person's social abilities and, when they make mistakes, to believe that they are behaving badly on purpose. How many times have you heard someone say, 'That person knows exactly what they are doing, and they are deliberately trying to wind me up!'

While it may feel like this to you, in fact it is rarely true. People with AS often struggle a great deal to get social things right. They cannot predict how their actions will affect others and therefore do not realise that they are getting things wrong or upsetting others until it is too late.

This guide is designed to help you understand people with AS. It explores the characteristics of AS and how these can affect everyday life. The workbook is designed to be interactive. It aims to increase your knowledge, but also challenges you to explore your own reactions to people with AS.

The workbook is not a diagnostic tool and should not be treated as a bible of AS; it is a starting point and should be used as a foundation for learning more about the person you support.

It can be used in several ways. It can be used with a working study group, concentrating on particular sections to learn more about the people you are supporting, or it can be used as a resource for everyday information seeking and problem-solving.

At the end of each section there is a trouble-shooting section with ideas about how to tackle problems. It is important that any ideas are discussed with the individual with AS and the team supporting them before being tried out. They should not be attempted by one person in isolation without reference to the individual's existing care plans.

A PERSON-CENTRED APPROACH

What is person centredness?

A person-centred approach is based upon learning what is important to the person you are supporting. It is about providing support that concentrates on that persons needs, abilities and desires. It is an empowering approach that encourages carers to gain a better understanding of the person they are supporting, and to assist them in achieving their own goals.

How is this relevant to the workbook?

This workbook attempts to give an overview of some of the characteristics that are common in the diagnosis of AS. However, it is important to remember that everyone with a diagnosis of AS is different.

It can be very easy when learning about a diagnosis and its related symptoms to forget that we are dealing with people. People who have:

- different life experiences

- different needs

- different desires

- different interests

- different thoughts, feelings and emotions.

It is extremely important that whilst using this workbook to learn more about AS we do not forget also to learn more about the person that we support.

Mathematically there are over 100,000 combinations of the symptoms that result in a diagnosis of AS. It is possible for two people with AS to have only one of these characteristics in common. This means that any two people who have AS may behave very differently; they are unique individuals and should be treated accordingly.

GETTING STARTED

To get the most out of this workbook, and to work sensitively with the person you support, it is important to find out as much as possible about them as a person first. The starting point is what they know and how they feel about their diagnosis of AS. While most people are relieved finally to understand how and why they are different from the general population, others are unhappy about the diagnosis. Some people just dislike being labelled, and some have not had a full explanation of what the diagnosis means. Others have not been told of their diagnosis at all. If you are going to try to work with someone to help them cope with their difficulties, they need to understand why their behaviour is seen as a problem. They need to have their diagnosis explained to them, unless there is an extremely good reason not to do so.

Before you begin, you should also seek the person you support's agreement for any exercises in the workbook that involve observation, and should seek their consent for any changes that you think about making to the way they are supported.

Once you have done all that, begin by completing the information sheet that follows, so that you have a record of all the important information about the person you are going to support. The sheet also has space for recording new things you have learned from completing the workbook.

Information sheet

Name: **Age:**

When was AS diagnosed?

By whom?

How old was the person when the diagnosis was made?

What was the process leading up to diagnosis? (e.g. Did it take a long time? Did they see a lot of different professionals? Were they misdiagnosed with other conditions first?)

Do they have other diagnoses as well (learning disabilities, mental health problems, physical health problems)?

What features of AS do they show?

How is their AS currently supported?

What new understandings did you find from using the workbook?

What new ideas for supporting them did you find using the workbook?

1 Understanding Other People

As they grow up, most people develop a sort of 'social radar' that helps them pick up on other people's thoughts, feelings and preferences. They do this without realising they have done it. People with Asperger syndrome (AS) find this very difficult and need help.

Exercise

Think about a person you know well. How do you know:

- when they are in a bad mood?

- what they would like for a gift?

- if they didn't enjoy a meal or a social event?

To decide these things you probably use a range of skills: reading body language, picking up hints, asking questions, putting yourself 'in their shoes'. People with AS find this difficult if not impossible. Problems understanding others' thoughts and feelings are often referred to as lacking 'theory of mind' or having 'mind blindness'.

People with AS may find it difficult to understand the following:

- other people's thoughts

- motivations (e.g. the reason why someone did something)

- intentions (e.g. what the person planned or meant to happen).

They often fail to notice how others feel:

- mood states (e.g. tired, ill, 'fed up')

- reaction to events (e.g. upset following a death)

- reactions to others' behaviour, including theirs (e.g. hurt feelings, boredom).

They are often poor at working out the wishes and preferences of others:

- things they want

- things they enjoy

- things they find interesting/boring/frightening.

Sometimes a person with AS may not consider other people's reactions at all, or may behave as if others' thoughts or feelings are the same as their own. This can make them appear insensitive, selfish or ungrateful. At other times it can make the person with AS vulnerable, because they fail to realise what is going on.

For example, the person with AS may mistake other people's teasing of them as overtures of friendship.

Mary enjoyed going bowling but was not very skilled. Her odd behaviour and colourful clothes made her stand out at the bowling alley. Some of the regulars would shout 'Here comes the champion!' when she arrived at the bowling lane. Mary thought they were praising her skill and was pleased to have made some new friends.

People with AS also often misunderstand the motivations of those trying to help them, mistaking their concern for interference.

> Tony lives alone, but doesn't manage well. His house is dirty and he looks thin and scruffy. A kind neighbour offered to come in and help him clean up the house. At first he was pleased that she was being friendly. However, he disliked the changes that she tried to make in his way of doing things and eventually he shouted at her and hit her. The neighbour complained to the police and Tony was arrested. He did not understand what he'd done wrong. Tony feels his neighbour was to blame as she interfered.

Another difficulty that can arise is that of not understanding changes in people's moods – someone with AS expects people always to be the same. If someone's mood changes they may not understand why, and become very upset.

> George's key worker, Andrew, was usually cheerful and enjoyed banter about Liverpool football club. One day Andrew had a bad hangover and would not join in. George became withdrawn and later tore up Andrew's Liverpool scarf. Staff finally discovered that George thought that Andrew did not like him any more.

Similarly, people with AS may not understand that a person is upset about something and needs comforting.

> Mandy had worked with Matthew for five years and often told him about her elderly mother. One day Mandy told Matthew that her mother had died. Matthew simply said, 'Has she?' and then asked when they were going shopping. Mandy was hurt and thought Matthew was callous. As the death did not upset Matthew, he could not understand why Mandy should be distressed. He could not imagine how she felt.

People with AS often do not understand other people's reactions to their behaviour.

> One day Tom was very angry and his shouting was frightening the other people in his house, so the care staff asked him not to go into the shared areas. Tom stopped using the lounge completely from then onwards, and became very withdrawn. The puzzled care staff finally realised that he thought he was not allowed in there because people did not like him.

The problems that people with AS have with understanding other people's likes and dislikes can lead to some frustrating but sometimes amusing situations. For example any gift a person with AS gives is more likely to fit with their own interests than those of the person receiving it. Or if they make a cup of tea for you, they may not ask you about milk or sugar but will make it how they would like it. However, when these things happen a lot it can cause serious tensions in shared living situations.

PROBLEMS THAT CAN ARISE IN A SHARED HOUSE

In a shared house people have to accept that other people do things differently. However, the person with AS will not understand this, and problems may arise in the following ways:

Food, snacks, drinks

- They expect everyone in the house to eat fish and chips just because they like it.

- They put sugar in everyone's tea regardless of choice.

- They eat all the ice-cream that was meant to be shared.

Household chores

- They don't do their share of the chores.

- They insist that chores are done the way that they would do them.

Listening to music

- They impose their taste in music, and the volume of it, on others.

- They are angry if others play music when they want to be quiet.

Watching a shared TV

- They turn over to their favourite programme regardless of the fact that others are already watching a programme.

Lights, windows, doors

- They impose their choice of temperature/lighting levels, etc. on others.

- They open windows or doors without reference to others.

Having to resolve such problems can cause a great deal of stress for carers who are supporting the person with AS, and for his house-mates. Even if the person with AS lives at home there can still be problems of this kind.

Darren lives with his mum at home. In the evening Darren's mum likes him to come and sit with her to watch television. He doesn't understand why she likes him to be there, and resents her wanting him to be. He gets cross and shouts at her when she tries to persuade him.

Even when others try to explain how they are feeling, the person with AS may find it difficult to understand. They will probably not be able to change their behaviour. This can make others feel hurt, upset or angry. The person with AS is often seen as ungrateful for the care and support they have been given, because they will not change.

Exercise

After getting their permission and consent, observe the person with AS who you support, and make a note of those situations where the person has misunderstood or misinterpreted others' feelings, thoughts or behaviour.

Do these problems occur with any particular people/activities/situations?

Is there any way that you could help the person to understand these situations better in the future?

✍ Understanding others – Trouble-shooting

Don't expect someone with AS to pick up hints – they won't. Always spell out things clearly. Say what you want or how you feel.

A person with AS is likely to be oblivious to things that seem obvious to you. For example, you will need to spell things out in the following ways:

- 'When you say I am fat, it makes me unhappy.'

- 'I have a headache today, so I would like you to turn your music down, please.'

- 'Your mum doesn't really like train timetables: I think she would prefer to have some flowers.'

Always try and explain your motivation for doing things to a person with AS. If you leave them to guess, they may assume that you are interfering or spying on them.

For example, they may worry about your writing notes about them, or want to see what you are writing about someone else. You will need to explain very clearly:

- 'I have to write notes about you and your day so that my bosses can check that I am doing my job properly.'

- 'I can't show you what I am writing – it's about someone else and they will be upset if I let you see it.'

You could use cartoon drawings to show more clearly how people feel in different situations. For example, 'Social Stories'™ (see Additional Reading and Information) are used to illustrate how people might behave in a particular situation. Using drawings or pictures with these can make them easier to understand.

You can write or draw profiles of special people in the person's life, which will help them to get a better idea of how they should behave towards that person:

- 'Your mum likes to keep in touch with you. She likes to get a card for Christmas. She likes it when you give her a present for her birthday.'

- 'Things your mum likes are flowers, chocolates and going to the cinema.'

- 'Mum does not like railway timetables, like you do. If you give her a railway timetable she will be upset.'

- 'If you give her something she likes she will be happy.'

If you have to criticise, or intervene over someone's behaviour, then make it clear that it was their behaviour that was not welcome, not them as a person. Try and add a positive comment as well:

'When you shout it frightens people, so I must ask you to go to your room. When you are calmer, everyone will be happy for you to join them in the sitting room again, because they like your company when you are not shouting.'

This gives a clear message about what is OK and what is not. However, you will need to keep doing these things. Do not expect the person with AS to learn or remember what others want or think. People with AS find this hard anyway, and they also have poor short-term memories, so they are likely to forget.

2 Communication

People with Asperger syndrome (AS) have a range of difficulties with communication. They may have the following difficulties in holding a conversation:

- starting a conversation

- saying 'yes' for a quiet life

- keeping up a conversation

- changing topic

- dominating the conversation

- interrupting and talking over people

- not knowing when the conversation has ended

- saying things at the wrong time

- taking things literally

- using long or formal words and odd speech

- using strange accents or emphasis

- saying things which they do not really understand, but which get a reaction.

All people with AS have some difficulties with communication. However, the types of problem they experience vary greatly. While some people don't know what to say, others seem never to stop talking.

STARTING A CONVERSATION

> *Exercise*
> Do you have an idol?
>
> Imagine that, at work one day, your boss tells you your idol has just arrived and wishes to come and speak to you.
>
> What would you say? How would you feel?

Although you might feel very scared and nervous, you would probably have some idea of how to start a conversation. These ideas are based on our ability to make judgements about the person we are with, our knowledge of them, and past experience of talking to others. For example you might ask David Beckham about football, America or 'Posh Spice'.

People with AS do not appear to be able to draw on this kind of knowledge. They are likely to experience every social situation as scary. In some cases people with AS can start a conversation reasonably well, but it soon becomes obvious that their communication skills are very limited. They may only be able to talk about one thing, or quickly run out of things to say.

SAYING 'YES' FOR A QUIET LIFE

Some people with AS learn that saying 'yes' can often end a conversation quickly. As a result they may answer 'yes' to a question in order to get someone to go away, rather than because they really mean 'yes'. This can lead to an outcome that is confusing and annoying both for the person with AS and the person asking the question.

KEEPING UP A CONVERSATION

Some people with AS hold a conversation as though they were following a script:

> Patrick starts every conversation with 'What colour is your front door?' Then he asks 'Are you married?' and follows up with 'How many children have you got?' He does not change this formula, regardless of the answers he gets.

People with AS find it difficult to understand that other people have their own thoughts, feelings and agendas. As a result they may not alter their conversation in response to what the other person is telling them. This can be confusing for others.

Exercise

Using the script below attempt a conversation with one of your work colleagues. Do not allow yourself to deviate from the script. Whatever your colleague says in response to your question, you must follow with the next line from the script:

1. Hello, how are you today?

2. Did you have a good journey to work?

3. How are your family?

4. What did you do last night?

How did it feel being tied to a script in the conversation?

How did the person you were talking to react to you?

You probably found this experience odd and frustrating. The script in the exercise can be very typical of someone with AS, especially those who are less able. They tend to ask lots of questions without listening or replying to the answers they receive. People with AS may not update their answers to people's responses as we would expect them to, and they often stick rigidly to their script.

CHANGING TOPIC

Many people with AS find a change of topic difficult.

> Talking to Alex about his CD collection began very well. We talked about his favourite girl group. Alex seemed to genuinely enjoy our conversation, and became very animated in the way he talked. I moved on to ask Alex what he thought about another girl group; he became very puzzled and repeatedly said that I was confused and didn't understand what he was trying to tell me. It was clear that he did not know how he should reply; the conversation appeared to stop dead.

The problem for people with AS is that conversation is unpredictable, with rather loose structures. Because they tend to think in fairly rigid ways, and like things to be predictable, they may be thrown when the topic changes. Conversation may seem quite easy when you are talking about their favourite topic, but will become hard work if you try and change to something else.

If you find that a person with AS repeatedly says things like 'you don't understand', this can be their way of telling you that they are confused and struggling with the conversation.

People with AS can have a good vocabulary and may appear to talk easily. It is easy to overestimate the abilities of someone with AS. Initially, a person with AS may appear to be capable of holding a good conversation. However, when talking to the person for a longer period of time their difficulties can become more noticeable. You may suddenly realise that you are having the same conversation over and over again!

DOMINATING THE CONVERSATION

Some people with AS are happy to talk, but tend to dominate and take over the conversation, only talking about what they want to talk about. Usually, when this occurs, the person gets carried away talking about a special interest they have. They will fail to notice that others are not so interested.

> George's younger brother, Craig, had just returned from seeing the new Disney film at the cinema. Excitedly, Craig tried to tell George about the film he had just seen and became very upset when George dominated the conversation by talking instead about his favourite subject, *Star Wars*. George had no idea that he had done anything to upset his younger brother, and could not understand why Craig no longer wanted to talk to him.

When a person with AS starts talking about their special interest, you may find it extremely difficult to:

- get them to stop talking and listen

- get away from them (waiting for them to stop doesn't work)

- tell them anything else

- find out anything from them.

The person with AS thinks that because they are enjoying themselves and finding the conversation fascinating, you must be too!

You may also find that the person with AS jumps from one topic of conversation to another without any logical connection between the two. This can make the conversation very difficult to follow, and in some cases can result in total confusion. There is a connection in their own mind which they do not think to explain to you. They just assume that you will know, because they do.

INTERRUPTING AND TALKING OVER PEOPLE

Imagine trying to have a conversation with someone else who talks repeatedly over you, insisting they be heard!

How would you feel?

As we grow up, we learn from our experiences that it is rude to interrupt or talk over someone else when they are speaking. This is a basic rule of conversation. People with AS do not learn this in the same way, and may insist on saying what they want to say, regardless of others. They do not appear to know there is such a rule. Others may be able to learn that there is a rule 'I must not interrupt', but are still unable to apply it in a real-life conversation.

Once again this is often because someone with AS cannot see things from another person's point of view. However, sometimes it may be the result of memory problems; they are afraid they may forget what they are about to say if they wait for others to finish their conversations first.

Jeff had been attending a friendship group for several months. When the facilitator asked another member of the group how their week had been, Jeff immediately started to tell the group what he had been doing, and on numerous occasions had to be reminded that it was not his turn to speak. Even when reminded, Jeff continued to interrupt. He found it very hard to stop himself.

People with AS have their own agenda, and fail to realise that other people have theirs. While some have trouble starting any conversation, sometimes you may find that the person with AS continually takes over. When this happens, they usually want to talk about their special interest, and nothing else.

NOT KNOWING WHEN THE CONVERSATION HAS ENDED

There are ways we signal the end of a conversation to each other. Small silences, changes in eye contact, slight movements away from the other person, stock phrases such as 'Well, I must be going...' and so on.

People with AS do not pick up these subtle cues that a conversation has ended. You may feel that your conversation has come to an end and attempt to walk away, only to find the person with AS following you, still talking. People with AS will often need clear and direct prompting or instruction that the conversation is finished.

Exercise

Over a period of one week (with the person with AS's permission and consent), note how many times they interrupt a conversation or talk over people.

Situation	What happened?

Note what it is that you think the person with AS is trying to convey – are they worried or excited about something?

Are they trying to tell you something that holds great value for them?

Each time, note how this behaviour makes you feel. Angry? Irritated?

Also note how you or others react to this behaviour.

Feelings	Reaction

Does the person with AS realise the effect of what they have done or said?

Impact on other person

It is easy when something is annoying to become overwhelmed with our own feelings and irritations. When working with someone with AS, it is important to think about whether their behaviour is intentional and what their motivation might be. Remember that people with AS find social situations very difficult. Something that we may find rude or annoying is usually unintentional.

SAYING THINGS AT THE WRONG TIME

People with AS lack some of the basic social skills that we take for granted. Most people are aware that to say what we are thinking or feeling, regardless, is not acceptable in many situations. To 'speak our minds' can be seen by others as odd, eccentric or, sometimes, rude.

People with AS do not have this awareness. Remember that we have already noted that they are unable to see things from another person's point of view, and have an obsession with their special interest. Together these difficulties mean that people with AS sometimes make mistakes by saying the wrong things at the wrong time.

> Tom lived at home with his elderly mother. Her best friend, Vena, visited every week, often close to the time that Tom's favourite TV programme was on. One day, when she had stayed longer tha usual, and the programme was due to start, Tom said to her, 'Aren't you going home yet? I think it is time you went.'

Tom had no idea that his mother or her friend would be upset by this remark. He was just honestly saying what was on his mind. This honesty means that people with AS may often say aloud, in public, things that others would only think. This can cause great embarrassment or sometimes just amusement.

> Louise likes to go to the supermarket to help with the weekly shopping. One day, when Louise is in the supermarket, she notices a bad smell. She approaches

a young man and asks him very loudly, 'Was that you that just farted?' The man looked shocked and hurriedly walked away in embarrassment, but Louise had no idea why he was upset.

People with AS will not pick up the signals that a social 'white lie' is called for. If you ever want an honest answer to 'Does my bum look big in this?' ask someone with AS!

The outcome does not always have to be disastrous, if people are able to use humour to see the funny side of things.

Exercise

What would be the reaction if you said the following phrases to people?

Phrase	Partner?	Work colleague?	Stranger?
'I love you.'			
'You've put on weight.'			
'What are you doing tomorrow?'			
'I've got a boil under my arm.'			
'This bus is a Routemaster 100 first made in 1965 by...'			
'I would love to see you naked.'			

TAKING THINGS LITERALLY

If I were to say to you, 'You need to pull your socks up', you would know that I meant that you should try harder, and improve what you are doing. People with AS have real problems with slang, figures of speech or sarcasm. If I said 'You need to pull your socks up' to an individual with AS, I would not be surprised if they bent over and pulled their socks up! People with AS take things very literally. They are also unable to understand sarcasm and often miss the point of jokes. They fail to notice the tone of voice that can change the meaning of a phrase.

> On leaving Mike's appointment I noticed that it was raining heavily. I said to Mike, 'Great! Just the kind of weather you want for driving on the M25!' Mike looked at me in a baffled manner and then began explaining that rain was dangerous for driving and could not understand why I should say I was pleased that it was raining.

Some common phrases can be very confusing to someone who takes things literally. What might these phrases bring to mind?

- 'It's raining cats and dogs out there.'

- 'Come on, get yourself in gear.'

- 'I'll take a rain check on that.'

- 'Make the bed.'

- 'You are driving me round the bend.'

- 'I'm snowed under with work at the moment.'

- 'Take no notice of her – her bark is worse than her bite!'

- 'It's no use crying over spilt milk!'

- 'You're cutting your nose off to spite your face!'

Imagine what these sentences might mean to someone with AS, who takes things literally. They could be extremely confusing and ambiguous if taken at face value. It is easy to forget this when talking to a person with AS and we may leave them feeling very confused or worried.

Exercise

Make observations of common confusing and sarcastic phrases used by you and colleagues when working with individuals with AS, over one week. Note down how often these phrases/comments are used, who says them, and in what context:

Idioms/ sarcastic comments	Who says them?	Context	No. of times

What did the person really mean in each case?

How could this be rephrased more clearly for the person with AS to understand?

USING LONG OR FORMAL WORDS AND ODD SPEECH

People with AS may have a good vocabulary, but tend to use more formal ways of speaking than most people. Sometimes they use unnecessarily long words and their choice of words can be unusual. They may pick up words from others that they will use without really understanding them.

> Martin was overheard telling another resident, 'I am going home for the weekend; I will be "on call".' It was obvious that Martin had no idea what this really meant, but he had heard his carers say it, and so copied it.

People with AS may speak in a very pedantic manner. They will often include all the information that is linked to what they are saying regardless of whether it is relevant or not. This can make conversation confusing and sounds odd.

> Talking to Julie about her forthcoming birthday, I asked what she might like as a present. She replied, 'My birthday this year is on Tuesday 7 March. I was born on Thursday 7 March in 1980, at 6am in the morning, at St George's hospital in Tooting, which is in London. I would like a new CD for my birthday, thank you.'

USING STRANGE ACCENTS OR EMPHASIS

You may find that some people with AS talk with an unexpected accent, e.g. they may adopt an American accent because they have heard it and like it.

SAYING THINGS WHICH THEY DO NOT REALLY UNDERSTAND, BUT WHICH GET A REACTION

People with AS, especially those who are less able, may sometimes use expressions that they have heard other people use, because of the reaction that they get. Usually they do not fully understand the impact of what they are saying.

> Pete hates people going into his room without permission. He recently threatened a member of staff who was going into his room to collect some dirty mugs. He said that if he ever found her in his room again he would 'slit her throat'. Pete did not really wish to hurt her but he had learned that saying this made people very unlikely to trespass in his room again.

Exercise

Make observations of your client over one week. Record attention-getting words or phrases that they use. Make a note of how and when they use this word/phrase:

Word or phrase   **Context**

Is it an appropriate word or phrase for them to be using in that context?

Do they understand the meaning of the word? Check by asking them.

If they do not understand the correct meaning, what meaning do you think the word holds for them?

It is important to be aware that although the person with AS may use long and complicated words, or ones that generate an emotional reaction from others, it does not mean they understand the meaning of the phrase or word they are using. It is important to explore their vocabulary with them and the meaning that such words or phrases have for them. Do not assume that it will be the same as it is for most people.

✍ Communication – Trouble-shooting

This section looks at how to cope with the problems that can arise when you talk to people with AS. Often they sound odd or different, and they may say things which seem rude, cruel or hurtful. You may also feel that they don't listen to you – they ask the same question over and over again, or seem to ignore what you have said. Carers and families often find this one of the hardest things to deal with. These problems are the result of the fact that people with AS have unusual brains. They are rarely being deliberately nasty; they are just unaware of others' feelings.

Starting a conversation and keeping it going

Teach the person with AS ways to start a conversation appropriately – how to ask questions politely, and how to listen to the answer given. You will really need to spell this out in detail for them.

For someone who enjoys games, explain to them that conversation is like a game of tennis; both parties have to take turns to play, or it doesn't work. Practise this with them, using the Rules of Conversation Worksheet at the end of this section as a guide.

It may help to teach the person a useful phrase to use when they are struggling, to help them out of an awkward situation, e.g. 'I'm sorry, I don't mean to be rude, but I need to go now.'

Saying 'Yes' for a quiet life

Do not just accept 'Yes' as the answer to your question, without checking that the person with AS has really understood. Ask them to repeat back to you what they really want.

Try to use open questions such as 'What do you want for lunch?' If this is too difficult for them, offer a choice: 'Do you want beans or cheese on toast?', so that it is not possible to simply say 'Yes'.

Changing topic

Again you may have to be quite blunt in explaining where the person you support is going wrong. Help them to understand that although they find their special interest fascinating, not everyone else will. Teach them some simple topics to talk about, such as the weather, or what they saw on TV, which they can use instead.

Dominating a conversation, interrupting and talking over people

This can be a difficult area. Make sure that the person with AS understands what you are trying to do. Often they will talk over others because they wish to talk about their favourite special interest. However, sometimes it can be because they are afraid they will forget what they want or need to say if they wait.

If they interrupt for fear of forgetting, try to find a way for them to hold on to the thought, e.g. by writing it down.

Explain, kindly but firmly, that interruptions and sudden changes of subject spoil the 'game' of 'conversational tennis'. Make it a rule of the game that you must allow someone else to finish speaking before you begin. However, you will probably need to remind them lots of times about this rule. They will forget that too!

Give them lots of praise (after the conversation has ended) when they manage not to interrupt or speak over someone else who is already talking.

Stop them immediately if they do interrupt or change the subject when someone else is speaking – then explain clearly why you are stopping them.

Overcome your inhibitions – politely but firmly say exactly what you want from them. If you need to go, and they keep on talking, then say so. They may even be grateful as they are unlikely to know that they are boring you.

In a group, it may be helpful to have a visual 'stop talking' card that can be held up so that the person with AS can see that it is someone else's turn to talk. Or you might try a 'stop talking' hand gesture that you have agreed with them earlier.

Do not rely on them to read your body language, or to pick up other cues that you are bored with the conversation. You will need to be blunt and use phrases such as:

'I have got to stop talking to you now. I must go back to my room and get on with some work.'

'Thank you for telling me about this but I am not going to talk about it any more now. You can talk to me about it for five minutes at 7.00pm. Now please think about what you have to do next.'

It may help to structure the conversation by writing things down, e.g.

'Today we need to talk about:

1. Topic X

2. Topic Y

3. Topic Z.'

Tick these off as you go. Keep the list where the person with AS can see it too, so you can bring their attention back to each topic if they wander, or when you finish the one before.

Saying things at the wrong time

If the person with AS wanders off the point, or interrupts with something inappropriate, this is often because they have not been able to follow the conversation that is happening around them, and their mind has wandered on to other things. Someone with AS finds it difficult to keep track of a conversation between several people. You can help them get back on track by saying something like, 'We are talking about [topic] at the moment.' If they are more able, you may be able to help by reminding them of what has been said, as briefly as you can.

If the person with AS says something that upsets you, such as 'You're late!' when you have been stuck in traffic and tried your best to get there on time, you need to try to explain to them both why you are late, and how it is sometimes unkind to point it out in such a way.

Use Social Stories™ to teach the person with AS how to tell white lies. You will need to explain clearly that these kinds of lies are only OK when they stop somebody's feelings being hurt.

Taking things literally

Try not to use sarcasm, or sayings like 'It's all swings and roundabouts', when talking to an individual with AS – you will just confuse them. Use simple phrases that say exactly what you mean.

Don't assume that the person with AS has understood what you have said. You may need to explain more than once, and go over it several times. Check back with them by asking them to tell you what they think has been said. This is true even for people who seem quite able.

It may be useful to make a list of common sayings, with simple explanations alongside, to help the person understand their meanings. Little pictures can help too. Make this into a dictionary that can be kept by the person with AS. For example:

'Throwing a wobbly!' means to become very angry and upset.

'Stop throwing a wobbly!' means calm down and don't get so upset.

Using long or formal words and odd speech

If a person with AS uses words or phrases in odd ways, it may be that these have a special meaning for them. It may be worth asking them a bit more about this. They may mean something different from what everyone else means when they say it. Some people will even have their own words for things.

Once you have discovered their own meaning, it might be useful to give them a way to explain this to others. For example:

'When I say... I really mean...'

If they say something that sounds odd or rude, gently tell them why, and explain what it might be better to say.

If they say something that is very worrying or scary, take the time to check out whether they understand what they have said and whether they really mean it before panicking.

If they are saying scary things to make things happen you will need to explain why that is not appropriate and try to find something else that gets the message across in an effective but less worrying way.

They won't be able to change quickly, and some people may not be able to change at all. Expect to have to say the same things many times.

Coping with your reaction

When you feel yourself reacting badly, think about why you reacted in that manner. It is important that you reflect on your reactions to people with AS. Their behaviour is not intentional, but sometimes others assume that the person with AS is 'winding them up'.

This is rarely the case. Often the person with AS is baffled as to why things they say get such a negative reaction, and this can make them distrustful of people.

Talk to your colleagues and share your feelings. Explore alternative ways of managing your reactions. Remember that much of what happens is the result of the difficulties that AS presents, rather than the person being deliberately awkward.

Example:

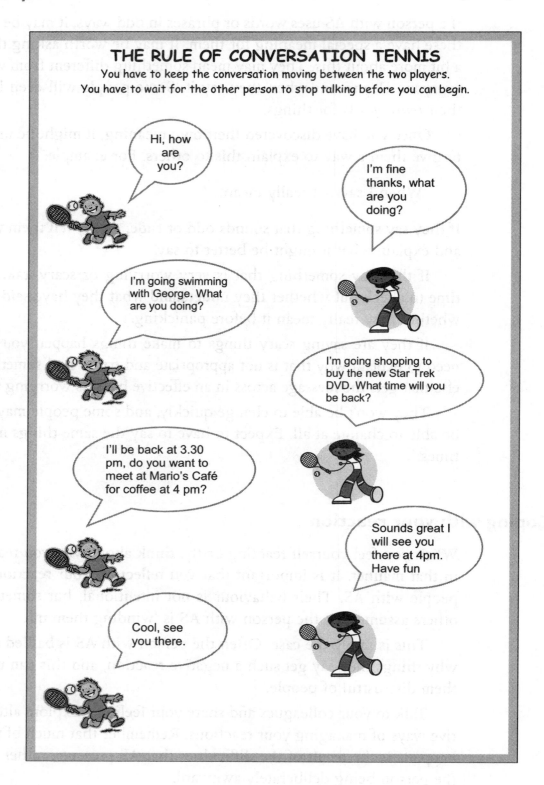

3 Odd social behaviour

People with Asperger Syndrome (AS) are often seen as odd. They behave in ways which are unusual to the rest of us. They have particular problems in understanding the social rules that exist around non-verbal behaviour, such as the following:

- standing too close

- inappropriate touch

- eye contact

- intimidating behaviour, such as following people

- pacing

- rocking.

STANDING TOO CLOSE

Someone with AS is not always aware that they are invading someone else's personal space. You may find that they lean over you when they talk to you or stand so close that they are touching you. They may behave in this way regardless of how well you know you.

This kind of behaviour can be quite unnerving and intimidating and may result in other people avoiding the person with AS. Women may find it particularly threatening, as close contact often suggests a sexual intention.

> ## Exercise
>
> How do you know when you are too close to someone?
>
> How close is too close for comfort?
>
> How do you know when you are invading someone else's space?
>
> What signals does that person give off?

It is very rare that people indicate that you are invading their personal space by saying 'You are standing too close to me, please step back!' They usually let the other person know by:

- moving away discreetly

- turning their back to the person

- looking downwards and trying to appear smaller.

People with AS are not able to pick up on these subtle non-verbal cues. It is likely that if someone steps away, the person with AS will take a step forward to get closer again.

> ## Exercise
>
> You will need two people. Stand opposite each other with about one metre between you. Take it in turns for one of you to move towards the other. Continue to move forwards a few centimetres at a time, until the distance between you feels uncomfortable for the person who is moving. Note the distance and then swap roles.
>
> - How did it feel standing one metre apart from the other person?

- How big was the distance between you when you began to find the experience uncomfortable?

- Was the distance the same for both of you?

- How did being too close make you feel?

Put yourself in the shoes of someone with AS. Imagine if you were not aware of the difference between standing one metre away from someone and standing so close that you are touching. This seems to be the case for people with AS. They are not aware of the socially acceptable distance that is usually kept between people. This can lead them to make mistakes when meeting people and can result in others feeling uncomfortable and avoiding them.

INAPPROPRIATE TOUCH

Exercise

Think about the person with AS who you are working with. Are there any situations when their use of personal space, or amount of touching, has been inappropriate?

- What happened?

- How did this make you feel?

- What did you do?

- How did they react?

Think about and plan three ways that you could help this person to become aware of this problem.

What would you do if a stranger approached you and touched you? You might be surprised, upset, angry or shocked, depending on how and where they touched you.

If someone strange touches us in an overly familiar way, our immediate reaction is to become defensive. Touch is an intimate way of communicating and is something that is bound by strict, but unspoken rules. These rules are affected by:

- where it happens

- the age/gender/abilities of the person involved

- the relationship between the two people

- familiarity.

The list is endless, and the rules are complicated. In addition they are not usually spoken about. We pick them up from our own experiences.

Look at how complex the following rules are:

Situations

On a crowded tube	it is OK to stand jammed against a stranger.
On a full bus	it is OK to approach and sit next to a stranger.
If a bus is half full	it is more acceptable to sit in an empty seat and you are less likely to sit with a stranger.

Relationships

Brother or sister	it is OK to touch your brother or sister and give them a hug.
Lover	it is OK to touch your lover intimately and in private parts.
Strangers	it is OK to shake hands but no other touch is usual.

A lot of these rules are unclear and ambiguous to many people, but people with AS find them even more confusing, or indeed may be quite unaware of them.

People with AS have been known to lean on strangers when talking to them, even pulling people's arms around as if they are something to explore or be played with. This is probably linked to their problems with realising how others feel. They are not aware that their behaviour can make others feel uncomfortable.

EYE CONTACT

Exercise

How do you feel if someone *stares* into your face?

- Intimidated?

- Unnerved?

- Embarrassed?

- Uneasy?

What do you think when you are talking to someone and they won't look you in the eye?

- Do you think that they are ignoring you?

- Are they being rude?

- Are they lying or being dishonest?

- Do you feel like you are talking to a brick wall?

People with AS have difficulty controlling eye contact. Sometimes they will avoid eye contact; they may not look at you at all or seem to look right through you. At other times the person with AS may stare steadily into your eyes. This can be confusing or frightening. It is often very difficult to interpret what someone with AS is signalling with eye contact. You may feel they are angry or want something from you, but this may not be the case. They could be signalling any of the following:

- They may be confused.

- They may be waiting for direction or prompting.

- They may want to talk to you but not know what to say.

- They may be concentrating on something else altogether.

Josh enjoys social contact and he has had some social skills training in the past, and he can tell you that eye contact is important. When Josh was introduced to his mother's friend, he spoke to her but looked at the wall. Sometimes he turned his face towards her while still looking away. It was clear that Josh had extreme difficulty with making appropriate eye contact despite knowing it was important.

Even when someone with AS knows what they should do, they may be unable to put this into practice, despite great effort.

Normal eye contact helps the flow of conversation. It is very difficult to keep up a conversation if someone does not look at you.

Exercise

Observe how the person with AS looks at you when talking to you:

- Do they stare?

- Do they appear to find it difficult to look at you?

Are these difficulties more noticeable in particular situations, activities or with certain people? Note which applies, if so.

What do you think the 'real' message of their eye contact is?

- How does it make you feel?

- How do you react?

- How does the person with AS deal with your reaction?

Now you've found out more about the problems around eye contact do you feel different about this?

Is there anything that the person might be able to learn to change and improve their eye contact?

INTIMIDATING BEHAVIOUR, SUCH AS FOLLOWING PEOPLE

How does it feel to be followed by someone strange?

- Scary?

- Unnerving?

- Worrying?

- Frightening?

It can be very intimidating to be followed by someone you don't know. All sorts of worries may go through your mind. It is human nature to want to know why the person is following us, and we naturally tend to assume the worst.

We have already seen that people with AS are not socially aware enough to know when they are invading someone else's privacy. In addition, they are not able to recognise when their behaviour upsets or unnerves others. Sometimes, when this is coupled with their tendency to take things literally and strictly follow rules, particular problems can arise. As in the following example, a person with AS may follow someone with the very best intentions.

Shaun followed a lady out of the supermarket to tell her that she had queued in the wrong aisle to pay. She had more than ten items but had queued in the 'Fewer than ten items' queue. Shaun was worried that the lady would get into trouble and thought it important that he tell her. Understandably the lady was worried when

Shaun followed her and she became quite frightened when he approached her. Shaun could not understand the lady's reaction. He was only trying to be helpful.

Sometimes the lack of social awareness can result in behaviour that is dangerous, illegal and frightening.

William has strong sexual feelings and will follow and approach anyone he likes the look of, for sexual contact. He is big and strong and will force his attentions on others. He is not fussy about who it is – male or female, young or old. He has often been in trouble with the police but doesn't seem able to control his behaviour. As a result he has had to live in a secure home for some years, although he does not understand why. Because he likes the sex, he assumes his victim will do too.

PACING

Pacing means walking up and down repeatedly in a straight line. You may notice that a person with AS tends to be agitated and nervous at times. One way that these feelings can show themselves is through pacing. Although harmless, others can find this very irritating.

Melanie held down a good job. However, her workmates complained that her walking up and down was driving them mad. Melanie did not know what else to do in her breaks. She was told she could walk up and down on the fire escape – out of sight of her workmates. This let her cope with breaks without upsetting her colleagues.

If pacing is a problem, it is important to think who it is a problem for, and look for practical solutions that will suit everyone, as above.

ROCKING

Another repetitive behaviour that people with AS exhibit when they feel agitated or nervous is rocking backwards and forwards.

> Ben, who has AS, often does a quick rock back and forth as he moves from one task to the next at college. His tutor was really surprised to see him do this as he seemed otherwise to be a very bright young lad.

So we have seen that people with AS, even those who may seem very capable in many ways, can also behave oddly. This can lead others to reject them as weird or odd, and may also lead to bullying.

✍ Odd social behaviour – Trouble-shooting

In many cases these odd behaviours will be very difficult to change. If behaviour is resistant to change and appears to be causing problems for the person with AS it may be advisable to seek professional assistance.

Invading personal space or inappropriate touching

Help the person with AS to have some understanding of what degree of touch or closeness is and isn't appropriate. This is complicated, as we have already seen, so they may find it difficult to remember. Try not to feel threatened by them; just remind them of the rules.

If a person with AS stands too near to you or to others, explain clearly and briefly why this is a problem:

> 'You are standing too close to me, and I don't like it. Please can you take a step back?'

It may be useful to talk about touch and body language in a role-play, rather than just dealing with the problem when it comes up. However, the person with AS may not remember what you have said. Using pictures may help.

If the person with AS finds it difficult to understand why this makes others feel uncomfortable, give them an example of something which might help them understand better:

'You know how meeting new people makes you anxious? When you stand very close to me it makes me feel the same. So please can you step back?'

A good practical exercise to teach someone with AS is to get them to hold out their arm with their fingers outstretched. If they can touch you, they are too close. It can be useful for them to do this with people while at home, but do not encourage them to do it with strangers, or this may cause more problems!

Make sure they have understood what is inappropriate and why. Get them to tell you in their own words. Demonstrate and role-play situations with them.

If they do the right thing at the right time, such as a good handshake, give them praise to let them know that they have done well.

If you feel that their behaviour makes them vulnerable to accusations of abuse, then seek professional help.

Eye contact

This is also likely to be very difficult to change. Explain to the person with AS that it is polite to look at others when talking to them, but not to stare all the time. Be patient, as they may not be able to get this right, even after being told.

You might find it helpful to teach the person a phrase to explain their behaviour to others:

'I'm sorry, I find it difficult to look at people – but I am listening to you!'

It might also be helpful to teach them to look at the other person's nose or mouth when talking. They may find this easier.

If they make a conscious effort to make eye contact but are still unable to do it well, it is still important to praise them for their efforts, so as to encourage them to keep trying.

Following people

Make sure that the person with AS understands why they should not follow people they do not know – you might find it helpful to use Social Stories™ with pictures to make this clear.

If this is something that you think puts the person or others at risk, it is important to seek professional help.

Pacing and rocking

Help the person with AS find a space where they can pace or rock, without upsetting or disturbing other people.

If other people are concerned by his pacing or rocking, explain why the person with AS needs to do this, and ask them to be tolerant.

Where to go for extra help

If problems persist and interfere with the person's everyday life it may be necessary to seek extra help and advice from professionals. The following can be good sources of specialist help:

- Psychology Services

- Community Team for People with Learning Disabilities (CTPLD)

- Adult Primary Community Mental Health Team (PCMHT).

For assistance in accessing these services contact the person's doctor. You may also find it useful to contact local voluntary organisations.

However, you should be aware that it can sometimes be very difficult to obtain services for a person with AS if they do not have a learning disability. AS is not a mental health problem and, unless the person also has a mental illness such as depression, the local mental health services may not offer help.

4 Need for Sameness

People with Asperger syndrome (AS) dislike change. Many of their unusual behaviours can be understood if you realise that they have a strong need for sameness:

- need for consistent structure and routine

- problems with change

- need for consistency in approach

- need for sameness in the physical and social environment

- putting things in order

- importance of rules

- problems with generalising rules

- repeated checking and repetitive questioning

- special interests.

NEED FOR CONSISTENT STRUCTURE AND ROUTINE

People with AS lack some of the basic social skills that most of us take for granted. The lack of these skills can cause anxiety for the person with AS, especially when they are exposed to a new social situation. It is extremely important for someone with AS to have consistency in their life and routines. This helps them to learn the social skills and behavioural strategies that enable them to cope with these situations.

PROBLEMS WITH CHANGE

If social rules and boundaries do not remain consistent, life becomes very confusing for people with AS. Their difficulty in understanding other people's thoughts and behaviour make new social situations particularly hard for them. This, in addition to their difficulties with making use of feedback, and problem-solving, causes great anxiety when situations, environments and people change without warning. They do not know what to do, or what is likely to happen.

NEED FOR CONSISTENCY IN APPROACH

A consistent approach to working with people with AS allows them to develop patterns of behaviour which enable them to cope. This consistency helps to build trusting relationships with the people who care for them.

Joe saw his psychologist about once a month to talk over his problems. He found it very worrying when he did not know when she was next coming to see him. He would ask the staff constantly about this, which they would find annoying. The psychologist solved this by giving Joe a year's worth of appointments, which they marked together in her diary and on his calendar.

Staff shortages or changes often mean that approaches to working with people with AS can be inconsistent. For example, a member of agency staff, who is unfamiliar with the person and their needs, may come into the person's home. This unfamiliarity is likely to make the person with AS feel threatened, and can lead to problems.

NEED FOR SAMENESS IN THE PHYSICAL AND SOCIAL ENVIRONMENT

As with people with autism, those with AS can find changes to their social and physical environment distressing. They may become unsettled by changes of staffing rotas, staff sickness, holidays and staff starting or leaving. They may also be distressed by physical changes to their home, workplace or local environment. This may range from minor changes of fixtures and fittings to redecoration.

PUTTING THINGS IN ORDER

Underwear and socks in the top drawer...tops in the third drawer... and trousers and skirts in the bottom drawer...

We all like things to be kept in a certain way. It keeps life familiar and manageable. We feel reassured that the space we are in is ours, giving us a sense of security.

Many people with AS also like things to be organised in a certain way, although their need for this is usually far greater than for most of us. Keeping things ordered can provide structure and predictability for people with AS. This behaviour is usually the person's way of coping with unpredictability and change in their daily life.

Keith lives in a home with ten other residents. He likes the furniture in the living area of the home to be arranged in a particular way. This often causes major problems between Keith and the other residents, and can lead to him becoming very distressed if they move it. He insists that the furniture be arranged as he likes it and cannot understand why this causes a problem for others.

From an early age most of us are encouraged to balance our needs against the needs of other people. We learn to make allowances for others.

People with AS have difficulty understanding that other people have their own needs. Therefore they don't really think about the needs of others, but just insist that they have things their way.

This need for order can cause problems in everyday life. In extreme cases it may be necessary to consult the relevant professionals (psychologist, psychiatrist) to rule out any additional diagnosis of obsessive compulsive disorder. It is often unclear at what point this need for order is so extreme, or irrational, that it becomes a mental illness.

IMPORTANCE OF RULES

Every social situation has its own set of rules and expectations, about what is OK and what is not.

- 'It is rude to interrupt.'

- 'You shouldn't talk to strangers about personal things.'

Social rules are often also specific to a country or culture. This can sometimes cause misunderstandings when we go abroad as the rules are different.

Some signs made with hands or fingers are different in different countries. What is a gesture of approval in one country can be an insult in another. If you do the wrong thing in a new country, you could get in trouble or offend people without realising. People with AS often have this experience in their own country. They do not realise what the rules are.

Most of us learn these rules while growing up and don't even think about them. They have become second nature to us, and we just picked them up as we went along.

People with AS do not pick up these rules while growing up. Their brains work differently and they don't pick up signals from other people unless these are very clear. They don't notice hints or tactful feedback about their behaviour, and sometimes don't learn even from quite forceful feedback like being shouted at or hit.

Unspoken rules about meeting a friend of your mother's for the first time are that it is polite to introduce yourself, and it is polite to make general conversation, asking questions such as:

- How did she meet your mother?

- What does she do for a living?

- Does she live nearby?

- Does she have children?

It is rude to use bad language in front of her, e.g. swearing or shouting.

It is rude to ignore her and go straight to your room.

It is polite to offer her a drink, such as a cup of tea.

It is polite to say 'It was nice to meet you', when she leaves.

It is unlikely that somebody sat you down and explicitly told you these rules. Most children are very tuned into the adults around them and quickly pick up when what they are doing is OK or not OK, because of the adults' reactions. They soon learn what gets approval and attention and what doesn't.

People with AS don't have this awareness of others. They don't pick up that they are getting it wrong unless the reaction is quite strong and direct, like being shouted at. Even then they may not realise what they did wrong, unless someone spells it out. They may just think the angry person is being unkind to them.

PROBLEMS WITH GENERALISING RULES

You may find that people with AS will stick to rules rigidly once they have been explained. This can cause other problems for them because they cannot judge that sometimes a rule might not apply this time.

> At a day service for people with learning disabilities, Susan was caught drawing on the wall in the lounge. She was sternly told off, and staff explained that it was unacceptable for her to vandalise the lounge in this way. Later that day Susan was in the kitchen where she began drawing on the wall again. Staff were dismayed by this behaviour and demanded an explanation. Susan explained that she knew she was not allowed to draw on the lounge wall, but that nobody had said she couldn't do this in the kitchen.

It is very important that when we explain social rules to someone with AS we take into account their tendency to take in only the literal meaning. We need to explore all the possible meanings of what we are asking them to do.

Exercise

Think about the person with AS who you support. Make a list of any odd or thoughtless things that they do.

Why do you think they do this?

What are the unwritten social rules that usually control this behaviour?

Does the person have any understanding of these rules? Or are they using the wrong rule? (Use the trouble-shooting section for ideas to help them learn these rules.)

REPEATED CHECKING AND REPETITIVE QUESTIONING

A common behaviour observed in people with AS is the repeated checking of times, activities or schedules.

Charlie punctuates all conversations with repetitive questions:

- 'What are you having for dinner tonight?'

- 'Where are you going when you finish here?'

- 'When am I going home?'

- 'When will it be Christmas?'

He will continue to ask these questions even when he knows the answers to them. This annoys his carers greatly. The following type of exchange is common:

Charlie: 'What are you having for dinner?'

Carer: 'What did I tell you last time you asked, Charlie?'

Charlie: 'You said chicken stir-fry!'

Carer: 'That's right, Charlie – that's what I am having for dinner!'

This behaviour can become so annoying that it would be easy to assume that the person is behaving in this way to 'wind you up'. However, this is very unlikely to be the case. Once you understand why they do it, it may be easier to bear!

- It may be that they fear change; the person checks on times and events to reassure themselves.

- Something is pleasant and the person wants reassurance that it will happen.

- Something is feared or dreaded, and the person wants reassurance that it isn't happening yet.

- They are checking out someone – do they give consistent answers? Can they be trusted?

- They want to get a response from someone.

- They have problems remembering.

Exercise

List any repetitive questions that the person with AS who you support regularly asks you or others:

What situations, activities or people trigger these questions?

What function do you think this serves for the person?

Are there alternative things that you can do to help or teach the person to do to meet this function without the repetitive questioning?

SPECIAL INTERESTS

It is natural for people to have things that interest them. Some people may have a favourite television programme, others may support a particular football team, and others may take great interest in music. However, people with AS tend to take things one step further.

How many people do you know that:

- know the local train timetable and are able to recite it?

- can tell you every character and every episode of *Star Trek* ever made?

- can name the make and serial number of every part of your computer?

Probably you answered 'none' or 'not many'. These areas of interest are very specific and thus unusual. People with AS have their own interests just like everybody else, but the difference is that their interests, like these above, can be quite unusual and detailed. They may be considered odd and eccentric by others. It is thought that over 90 per cent of individuals with AS have a special interest. These behaviours may serve an important purpose for the person with AS:

- They may be a source of genuine enjoyment and occupation.

- They may help the person cope with anxiety or stress.

- They give them something to talk about.

Robbie is very, very interested in soap operas on TV. He watches them all, and knows all the storylines and all the characters. He can tell you the number of each house that every character in *Coronation Street* lives in. He is keen to be friends with everyone, and thinks that they will share his interest. Whenever he meets someone new, he starts to tell them in great detail about all his favourite soap stories. He doesn't let them get a word in, and can't understand why people afterwards avoid him. He is hurt that they don't want to be friends any more.

For people with AS, their interests are special because they tend to be fascinated by the subject to the point where it is all they can think and talk about. Sometimes, in cases like the example above, where the interest is one that many people seem to share, the individual may become preoccupied with a particularly obscure aspect.

This tendency to talk endlessly about their favourite topic can be extremely frustrating for the person trying to hold a conversation with them or trying to get them to do something. These interests are often so intense that they may be referred to as obsessions. The person is likely to devote a tremendous amount of time to finding new information and facts about the subject, which may limit the amount of time they have to spend on other activities. However, it is important to realise that people with AS find their special interests a source of genuine enjoyment, security and comfort.

In some cases the person with AS may use the interest as a way of escaping from reality. If this is the case, you might notice that they spend more time on their special interest in times of worry or stress. In some cases special interests can become such an obsession for the person that their behaviour may become truly compulsive. Compulsions are explored more fully in the chapter on mental health problems.

Exercise

Over a period of one week, pay close attention to how many times the person you are working with refers to their favourite interest. Keep a diary of this, noting the date and time of each occasion.

What was the conversation?

On each occasion, make a note of how you felt about this conversation.

How did your reaction affect the person with AS?

Could you manage your reactions better in the future? How?

✎ Need for sameness – Trouble-shooting

Here are some ideas and suggestions to help you and your client cope with the need for sameness. Often this can't be changed but some of these ideas may make it easier to manage. If these tips are not successful in resolving the issues it may be necessary to seek professional help.

Need for consistent structure and routine

Develop a timetable of daily events with the person you support. Where the person has free time indicate this on the timetable. It may help to list a few things that they like and could do in their free time. For example:

Day	Morning	Afternoon	Evening	Nighttime
Mon	Swimming	Free time	Cinema	Sleeping
Tue	College	College	Free time	Sleeping
Wed	Ramble	College	Pub	Sleeping
Thurs	Shopping	Library	Phone Mum	Sleeping
Fri	College	College	Asperger group	Sleeping
Sat	Chores	Visit friends	Free time	Night club
Sun	Lie in	Swimming	Barbecue	Sleeping

Free time: listen to music, sort CD collection, have a coffee with a friend

These activities may not apply to the particular person that you support, but the example gives some idea of the way you could lay the timetable out.

You may also wish to include more details, such as:

- exact times of each event

- where they will be going

- who will be taking them there

- who will be bringing them back

- will they be going alone?

- will they have a coffee and a cake after swimming? who with?

To make the timetable more specific to your client you may wish to use pictures of them doing the actual activity.

People with AS often find it very hard to think of things to do without help. They may stick to one or two activities because they can't think of anything else.

A timetable provides a visual reassurance about what is going to happen, and when (perhaps also where). It should be kept somewhere it can be consulted at any time by the person when they feel anxious. Ideally it should be on a bedroom wall or, for more independent individuals, a foldable copy kept in a wallet/purse/bag.

You could also provide a pictorial staff rota for each week so that the person with AS knows who they will be working with and on which days. You may need to assess their reaction to this. Some people may become even more upset about staff changes if they are not on the plan. Others may be upset at seeing how long it is until their preferred member of staff is next on duty.

You could also provide a calendar or diary to show less frequent events, such as visits home to see family, birthdays, parties and visits to the doctor or dentist.

For less able individuals you may wish to use an alternative way of explaining when something is happening. If the person has to go to the doctor in two weeks' time, it may be useful to explain two weeks in terms of 14 sleeps. A chart can help with this so that the person can monitor how far away the event is by crossing each sleep off daily.

Try and ensure that wherever there have to be changes to the schedule, routine or staffing, that these changes are planned in advance and the person knows exactly what will happen.

If there is a sudden change because of sickness or an emergency, take time to explain slowly and clearly what is going to happen.

However, it may not be a good idea to tell the person too soon, as this can increase anxiety and may provoke repetitive questioning. Careful record keeping about the amount of notice given when a change happens, and how they coped, can help you to work out the right amount of notice to give them next time.

In either case, take your time to explain in simple language and short sentences what has changed and what will happen. Use visual cues to help, such as pictures of staff in cases of changes, or simple written notes.

Give the individual structured time to ask questions or voice any concerns that they have, and *give them time to adapt.*

Need for sameness in the physical environment

Be aware that the person you support may react to even very small changes to the physical environment. For some people, even a different wattage in the light bulbs, or the angle that blinds are adjusted to, will be noticeable. Think before you change *anything*.

If the person with AS becomes upset for no apparent reason, check carefully to see if any changes have been made to their environment.

If there has to be a change, then plan it carefully. Make sure that any major changes such as redecorating happen as quickly and smoothly as possible. Buy all the materials and fittings *before* the work starts, to minimise the length of time that things will be disrupted.

Wherever possible involve the person in the planning and decision-making. They may like to be involved in making the change, such as by helping with the painting, or may prefer to go somewhere else, such as on holiday, and return when the work is finished.

Make a note each time that you have major changes what approaches helped the person, and what did not. Major changes are usually infrequent, and it is easy to forget. Or you may have moved on to another job, and the new carers will not know the approach you used.

Staff changes are inevitable, but it can help the person with AS to adjust if they are managed in a consistent way. Give enough time for them to adjust to the news, e.g. two weeks. Explain why the person is leaving. This might be for a promotion, or to be nearer their family. Make it clear that everyone will miss the person who leaves.

It may be helpful to make an occasion of the leaving, by buying a present and card, and going for a nice meal out.

It might also help to make a memory book with a picture of the member of staff who is leaving, and what the person will and will not miss about them. For example 'Paul worked with me from April 2006 to July 2008. He left to train as a teacher. Paul told very funny jokes but he made terrible tea.' You could add to this for each person who leaves.

People with AS can find it difficult to cope with new members of staff. They may find it hard to trust a new person and worry that the person does not know what they need. It can be helpful for new staff to have access to a 'passport' about the client. This is a short document with key information about the person's likes and dislikes and how best to get on with them. This avoids new staff accidentally 'putting their foot in it' and making a bad start.

If the person with AS has strong preferences for certain staff members it can be helpful to observe how they interact with them. The preference may be based on patterns of behaviour, e.g. tone of voice, body language or style of communicating, that other staff can replicate.

For unexpected changes, such as sickness, make sure that the person is given precise and accurate information, e.g. 'Louise has flu and can't make it today. Gary will be here this afternoon. Louise hopes to be well enough to work on Saturday.'

If the sickness is longer term, and it is not clear when the person will be back, it may help if the client is encouraged to send a get well card and flowers.

Putting things in order

- Ensure that the person with AS has some control over how things in their life are ordered.

- Ensure they have one area or space (e.g. their room) in which they are able to exert total control over their life.

- If there is a reason why things have to be ordered in a way that they find distressing, ensure that time is taken to explain explicitly why this is necessary.

- It may be useful to write explicit rules about what is and what isn't acceptable so that they can refer to these later on.

Understanding rules

When the person with AS is entering a new social situation, it may help if you spell out for them, in advance, the social rules specific to that situation. You could write these down simply for them. Make sure they are aware what these rules and expectations are before they go. Use simple, short sentences in both speaking and writing.

Be sure to take into account that social rules may change very subtly in different situations. People with AS are unlikely to pick up on these differences. Consider these two different examples of eating out:

Pub	Restaurant
Find a table and note the table number.	Be aware that in popular restaurants you may need to book in advance.
Choose what you want to eat from a menu/blackboard.	Wait near restaurant door to be seated by waiter.
Approach the bar and wait to be served by the bar tender.	When seated look through menu and choose what you want to eat.
Order food and drink from the bar and tell them your table number.	Wait for the waiter to approach you to take a drinks and food order.
Pay bar tender for food and drink. Take drink.	When the waiter arrives place your order.
Collect cutlery etc. on way back to table.	Wait for the food and drink to arrive while sitting at the table.
Sit at table and wait for food. Enjoy drink.	Drinks usually arrive first, followed by the food.
When food arrives eat.	When food arrives eat.
When finished eating you are free to leave.	When finished eating ask for the bill.
	Wait for the bill to be brought to the table.
	Pay the bill and wait for the receipt.
	You may wish to leave a tip.
	You are free to leave.

These differences are small, and in some pubs or restaurants may be different again. If you have desserts afterwards, there are additional parts to the sequence, which makes it even more complicated. You will need to be familiar with the venue and teach the person with AS the correct sequence before they go. Rehearse the correct behaviour by role-playing with them.

Use Social Stories™ to help them understand the expectations of the new social situation, and encourage them to be confident enough to say 'I don't know' or 'I need help' in a situation where they are confused or stuck. It might help to identify someone that they could approach if this happens.

Repeated checking and repetitive questioning

There are a number of reasons why these behaviours might arise. Try to find out the reasons for questions, and then choose the appropriate approach:

Fear of change – Keep answering questions with a reassuring voice. Look for sources of stress, e.g. have things been changed without the person with AS being told?

Looking forward – Use a visual calendar for things that are being looked forward to. Let the person cross each activity off daily. Remove any activities as they are completed so that the person gets a sense of progress.

Worrying – Be supportive, and reassure the person. Look for ways to make them less worried. For example, remind them of times when things went well in the past.

Ways of interacting – Teach the person other ways of keeping a conversation going without asking the same questions over and over again.

Trust – Make sure you always give consistent answers, and don't be tempted to change them unless absolutely necessary. Keep to the same wording and look for other ways to reassure the person that you are reliable.

Set limits to let the individual with AS know how many times you are willing to answer the same question. It may help to write down the answer for them. You may also find it helpful to look at ways of helping them remember information that is important to them. Try to divert them to another activity they enjoy.

Special interests

Make sure that the person with AS is given time to spend talking about or investigating their interest. This could be added to their daily timetable.

Consider ways in which the interest can be used positively, such as in further study, drawing, making social contacts with others, or even obtaining employment.

Vary the way the interest is explored, e.g.:

- going to the library to do research

- using an internet café to do research

- joining a club where others have similar interests

- writing about the subject

- drawing pictures of it.

This can help to keep their daily life varied but still allows their special interest to be central to it. Brainstorming with colleagues may help you to think of other suitable ideas.

If special interests begin to become intrusive the following ideas may help:

- Look for things that may be unsettling the person with AS – if they are happy and occupied they may have less need to retreat into their special interest.

- If the behaviour is being used as a coping mechanism for stress, talk about strategies for dealing with stressful situations.

- Set limits – you may be able to agree that the behaviour can only take place for a certain length of time or in a particular place. It may be possible gradually to reduce this.

- Try to explain to the person with AS how their behaviour affects others.

- You may wish to use role-play/pictures so that they can understand how their behaviour affects others.

- Never try to get rid of a behaviour. Always attempt to build a better alternative, otherwise the person may replace the behaviour with something worse.

Staff stopped Simon from collecting newspapers as they cluttered up his room too much. Simon then switched to collecting crisp packets – these took up less room but smelt terrible and were unhygienic.

5 Memory and Attention

People with Asperger syndrome (AS) have problems with their short-term memory, or attention. They often have very good long-term memories, so they may be able to tell you in detail about something that happened to them five years ago, but not be able to repeat what you have just said. How can this be?

It happens because the two kinds of memory work very differently. It may make it clearer if you call short-term memory 'attention' and long-term memory 'memory'. In order to get something into long-term memory, you have to first pay attention to it. If you don't attend properly to something, you don't remember it.

People with AS have great difficulty in keeping their attention on one thing for very long. Even with their special interest, they may have to have breaks. Often their habit of going over and over the things they are interested in is their way of remembering what they want to remember. We all do this to some extent.

Exercise

Imagine you are in a crowded nightclub with loud music, people dancing around you and pushing past you. Someone tries to give you a mobile phone number, but you have nothing to write it down on.

How easy would it be to remember the number? What would you do to try to recall it? For people with AS, everyday life can feel very much like this situation.

Problems with attention contribute to all of the following:

- repetitive questioning

- distractibility

- rigid, unimaginative thinking

- difficulty with problem-solving.

People with AS often have very good long-term memories for times, dates, events and facts. Some are able to remember very specifically what they were doing a long time ago.

> Pete was asked, 'How long have you known Lee?' He replied, astonishingly, 'I met Lee on 21 July 1989, which would have been 15 years 2 months ago.'

This ability can cause problems for people with AS. They have good long-term memory, but when they can't remember what they were told five minutes ago, people assume that they are being deliberately difficult. However, their difficulty is actually linked to problems of attention.

REPETITIVE QUESTIONING

People with AS have the tendency to repeatedly ask the same question, over and over again. Sometimes, if you are on the receiving end, it can feel as though they are deliberately trying to annoy you. In some cases they may not only repeatedly question you, but you may hear them repeat a phrase or statement to themselves over and over again. This helps them to remember it.

> Steven talks to himself. He finds this comforting and it helps him to remember what he has to do. If someone asks him to do something, he will repeat the instruction over and over again to himself, as he goes to do it, so

that he doesn't forget. People sometimes think that he is mad because he talks to himself, and so avoid him.

Repetition keeps information active in the person with AS's mind, and enables them to remember what to do next.

Problems with attention make it hard for the person with AS to hold a conversation. They may forget what has just been said, so lose the thread of the conversation, and they may rejoin it with something completely irrelevant. Sometimes they forget what they have said themselves, and hence repeat themself. This kind of repetition in conversation can leave others feeling ignored and frustrated. People may feel hurt and irritated that the other person seems not to be paying attention to them and this can lead to a breakdown not only of the conversation but also of any potential friendship.

Problems with attention can also lead to the person with AS urgently interrupting others, to share some information that does not seem important enough to justify the interruption. This usually happens because they are afraid that if they wait for you to finish, they will have forgotten what they needed to say.

It is important to be aware that this behaviour serves an important purpose for the individual with AS. It can help them to remember what they need to say or do, or to remain focused on what they are doing. They are not doing it to be annoying and irritating.

DISTRACTIBILITY

People with AS have trouble keeping their attention on one thing. They are easily distracted from whatever they are doing. Because they have trouble keeping their attention on one thing, other things will grab their attention, so that they lose track of what they were doing. This can mean that important things are forgotten, like locking the door, or turning off the gas. As well as being potentially dangerous, this can be annoying to others, who feel the person is being careless, or deliberately difficult.

Mark's mother asked him to go to the front room to get a vase for the flowers. Mark returned five minutes later without the vase. Angrily his mother asked him, 'What did I ask you to get, Mark?' Mark had no recollection of his mother asking him to get a vase. He had been sitting watching the television when she asked him, and so not really giving his attention to what she said. As a result, he had only remembered part of it.

This loss of attention can be a problem even when the activity is something that the person with AS really enjoys, as in the example below.

Patrick finds it difficult to concentrate on the same thing for long periods of time. His favourite pastime is drawing; however, he finds it difficult to concentrate on drawing for more than five or ten minutes at a time before he needs a break. Once Patrick has had a break, he often has to take a couple of minutes to refocus on what it is he is drawing. Then he is able to relax and enjoy drawing again for another short period of time.

RIGID, UNIMAGINATIVE THINKING

People with AS often find it hard to learn new ideas or ways of doing things. This can lead individuals to become very fixed in their way of thinking. Part of this is because they find it difficult to solve problems if faced with anything new. If your attention is poor, it is hard to problem-solve because there are too many things to think about at once. You might find the person with AS seems stubborn and inflexible both in their behaviours and in what they can or will talk about. However, this is protective because, by being rigid, they don't have to cope with anything new. If they are forced to change for some reason, this can make them very anxious.

Elaine always goes to the shops on a Monday, to buy her groceries for the week. She becomes very anxious and upset when any Monday is a bank holiday in case she cannot do her shopping. She will often ask anxiously, 'Is Monday a bank holiday?'

DIFFICULTY WITH PROBLEM-SOLVING

To be able to solve new problems, we need to be able to attend to what is important, and hold it in our memory long enough to come up with an answer. If you have problems of attention you will find it hard to do this, so that you never get to the point of being able to decide what to do. Think about how difficult it is to solve a problem if you are very tired, or perhaps drunk! This is how it feels for people with AS all the time.

James gets the bus to work every day. One day the council dug up the road near his house where he regularly crossed the road. James did not know what to do, and became very anxious and upset. He had to go back home and ask his parents what he should do, in order to get to work.

Most of us, when our normal routine is disturbed, are usually able to think of an alternative. This is something that we take for granted. People with AS struggle to come up with alternatives when their routine is disrupted. This can cause major distress, upset and worry. This is the reason people with AS like sameness and routine. It helps them to feel that the world is safer, and more predictable.

When the person with AS is faced with something new, or the possibility of change, it may help to talk about this in advance and suggest alternatives. It is a good idea to write the ideas down somewhere safe, for the person to keep, e.g. in a diary or special notebook.

✍ *Memory and attention – Trouble-shooting*

Dealing with repetitive questioning

We have seen that this can arise for several reasons. If the person is forgetting what is said, try the following:

- Speak in short sentences with simple, clear language.

- Check that they have heard what you have said.

- Ask them to tell you what you said.

- Repeat to them if necessary, and check again that they have heard and understood.

- It may help to write things down for them. Make sure you write in short, simple sentences.

- Try to be patient.

Distractibility

- Do not expect someone with AS to concentrate for long periods.

- Allow them regular short breaks from whatever task they are doing.

- Encourage them to keep a notebook or diary and to note down what they are going to do, and what they need to remember.

- If they forget, encourage them to refer to their notebook or diary.

- Plan and organise everything you need before starting a task with someone with AS.

- Use visual cues to prompt the correct sequence for tasks.

- Reduce distractions, e.g. turn the TV off before doing the cleaning.

- Take five minutes at the beginning of the task for them to note down and talk through any concerns (such as worries that might be getting in the way of them being able to concentrate).

Rigid, unimaginative thinking

- Describe a situation to them, and then brainstorm alternative responses. If they prefer to use visual cues, you could try using Mind Maps or drawings.

- Give lots of praise when they successfully come up with alternative solutions.

Difficulty with problem-solving

- Brainstorming, as above, can help to develop problem-solving skills.

- For everyday activities, have a routine that the person with AS understands and stick to it.

- Identify activities that if changed unexpectedly would leave them worried and confused.

- Role-play alternative solutions with them that could be used in these situations.

- Encourage them to ask for help when they need it.

- Provide them with the name and number of someone that they feel comfortable to approach when they are struggling to think of an alternative in a problematic situation.

General tips

- Encourage the use of lists, diaries, calendars and visual cues.

- Try to be patient and make allowances for the AS person's problems with attention.

6 Daily Living Skills

Many people with Asperger syndrome (AS), even the most able, have problems coping with daily living. Problem areas may include:

- eating

- personal hygiene

- clothing

- daily routines

- looking after the physical environment

- sleeping

- managing money.

The difficulties that people with AS have that contribute to these problems include:

- lack of motivation for tasks that do not interest them

- poor organisation, planning and problem-solving

- poor attention and sequencing

- lack of understanding of how their behaviour affects others

- hyper/hypo-sensitivities

- rigidity and obsessionality.

People with AS often have problems with personal hygiene, daily routines and managing money. However, until these problems result in severe consequences for the person they may think that they are coping well and not be aware that anything is wrong. Their behaviour may appear confusing and contradictory to other people. For example a person with AS may refuse to wash themselves but be meticulous about cleaning the kitchen sink.

When other people try to help with any of these problems, the person with AS may think that they are interfering and become angry, hurt or upset. The following section aims to identify some of the problems people with AS may have in relation to everyday living skills.

EATING

The need for sameness may lead someone with AS to eat a very limited diet.

> George did not trust anyone else to prepare his food. He shopped for this himself and kept the food in his room. This caused several problems. He gained weight as he was eating too much, and became unwell because his diet was not balanced. The food he bought often went bad, as he had no fridge in his room, so he was at risk of food poisoning, too.

People with AS may also apply a routine to their eating pattern, which once adopted is very difficult to change, e.g. only eating pizza on a Wednesday night.

> ### Exercise
>
> Imagine you are visiting a foreign country and you are offered the local delicacy. This might be something such as:
>
> - dog/cat meat
>
> - snake
>
> - wood ants
>
> - grubs.
>
> Or imagine how you might feel if all your food was dyed blue. What would you do if there was nothing else to eat? People with AS can feel very strongly about what they want to eat and what not, and will refuse your offer of things they don't like. In the same way, you might refuse the foods listed above.

Choosing a very limited diet may relate to having an over-sensitive or under-sensitive sense of taste. Depending on how their taste is affected, they may insist on eating strong-flavoured spicy foods, or very bland plain foods. This may appear just picky or fussy, but it is usually the result of the sensory sensitivities. These are common in autism, but can also be associated with AS.

Insistence on a very limited diet can cause further problems if the home is shared with others. However, it is important that people have choices, and as long as their diet is balanced, even if it is unconventional, then they will not suffer harm.

Some people with AS may be highly distressed by a disliked food being on their plate even if they are not expected to eat it. Others can be very sensitive to how food is presented on the plate, for example, refusing to eat it if the different foods come into contact with each other.

Sometimes people with AS have problems with when to eat and how much to eat; they may want to eat at odd times, or may over- or under-eat. Women with AS may appear to have an eating disorder, but this is not the usual type of eating disorder, and is much more to do with their AS. However, there is some research that suggests that women with AS are more likely to develop a true eating disorder too.

> ### Exercise
> With the agreement of the person you support, keep a diary of what they eat for two weeks. Record not just the name of the dish, but details such as when they eat and where. Also note down the colour and texture of the food, and how it is presented. Look at the diary and consider:
>
> - Is their overall diet balanced?
>
> - Is there a pattern to what the person will or won't eat?
>
> - Can you identify any common themes (e.g. colour of food, types of food, times and places to eat)?

PERSONAL HYGIENE

People with AS sometimes have problems with managing their personal hygiene. Problem areas can be:

- forgetting to wash or disliking water

- forgetting to bath or shower or cleaning only certain parts of the body

- not washing clothes

- not brushing hair and/or refusing to have hair cut

- not brushing teeth and/or having bad breath

- not using deodorant

- not shaving

- for women, problems with managing periods.

Despite being able in many ways, Emma had great difficulty remembering what to do when she had a period. Her mother solved the problem by giving her a special bin to put the soiled pads in, and a picture sequence showing how to change and dispose of sanitary towels when she had her periods. This reminded Emma what to do, and completely solved the problem.

Most of us learn to wash and change our clothes regularly so that we do not smell unpleasant and upset others. People with AS are unlikely to think about this.

Edward always smells. He does not wash his clothes, although he is quite capable of doing so. Edward is very disorganised and just forgets to wash, as he is too absorbed in his hobby during his spare time. He needs someone regularly to remind him to wash his clothes, take a shower, shave and brush his teeth.

Most people learn to look after their clothes and appearance from quite early in life. People with AS may have never learned, or may be forgetful. Sometimes they do not feel a need to look after their appearance or personal hygiene. They may need constant reminding about keeping clean, changing their clothes, etc.

Being dirty or smelly are things that people with AS may be bullied or teased about. Taking care of these everyday problems may make their life much more manageable, and can help them to make friends, too.

CLOTHING

Even if clothes are kept clean, other problems may arise. These include:

- refusing to change clothes

- refusing to wear new clothes

- wearing the wrong clothes for the weather or occasion

- eccentric choice of clothes or lack of dress sense

- insisting on wearing the same colour all the time.

Some of these difficulties can relate to hypersensitivities – clothes can feel and smell very different when new or after being washed. People with AS may be sensitive to different fabrics or textures and prefer comfortable clothes, rather than caring what they look like.

Although at one level they do not think about what others think of their clothes, repeated comments about their clothing may feel like a personal attack. This can lead to problems, too.

DAILY ROUTINES

People with AS have great difficulty organising themselves and following sequences. We have already noted that they are distractible, and have problems of attention. When faced with a lot of demands, they will tend to get confused by all the different tasks that need to be done. Often they just give up and do none of them.

> Robert lived in a house with three other people. One of his fellow tenants asked for help because Robert was sleeping in the living room. The care manager was amazed when she found his room so full of rubbish that it was not possible to open the door. Robert had moved into the living room because he could no longer get into his bedroom.

The person with AS may have problems remembering to do these tasks, or may just not be able to organise themselves to do it. What seems to others a simple task such as 'tidy up your room' may to a person with AS seem completely overwhelming. You will need to break a job like this down into easier parts, such as:

- make the bed

- put your dirty clothes in the washing basket

- put your clean clothes away in the wardrobe

- put the rubbish in the bin

- empty the rubbish bin

- clean the washbasin

- vacuum the floor.

Sometimes the problem is that the person is unable to develop any kind of routine. They do things in the wrong order or get distracted and forget to do certain things.

Nicholas would get up at any time between 8am and lunch time. Sometimes he would bathe, but then put dirty clothes back on or leave shampoo in his hair. Nicholas sometimes forgot his internet sessions, which were booked at the library, and would get very angry when this happened. His carers worked with him to make visual reminders for his activities, e.g. a list on the bathroom wall to remind him to wash, shampoo and rinse his hair, and then to put on clean clothes. Together they planned a daily routine and drew up a timetable. Nicholas's carers woke him each morning to ensure that he got started on time.

Exercise

Look at the daily chores listed below:

- Do the laundry.

- Do the shopping.

- Put out the rubbish.

How many tasks are involved within each of these chores?

What would happen if you missed out a task or did them in the wrong order?

Keep a record for one week of the times you have to remind the person with AS that you work with to do something. Use these headings:

Day/Time   Task forgotten   Reminder   Outcome

Look at the record to see if there are any patterns.

Why do you think the person needs reminding to do these tasks?

Working together, can you identify ways to support them to be more independent?

LOOKING AFTER THE PHYSICAL ENVIRONMENT

People with AS often struggle with daily tasks. However, when it comes to less frequent tasks, such as weekly or monthly ones, they may completely fail to think about them. They may be unaware of the need to look after the house or appliances. When things go wrong, it may not occur to them to ask for help.

> Gordon had got in a muddle with his finances and his care manager visited him at home to try to sort out his benefits. She was shocked to see water running down the living room wall, and from the state of the carpet realised that this had been happening for some time. When she asked Gordon if he had informed the landlord he was surprised and said that he had moved his things out of the way, but did not realise that he should do anything else.

SLEEPING

Sleep can be a problem. Some people with AS do not follow the usual patterns of sleeping and waking. Others stay up to enjoy the darkness and quiet of the nighttime when others are asleep.

This can lead to all sorts of strange sleeping patterns. The person may stay awake all night and then fall asleep during the day. Or they may oversleep in the morning, not wake up till late, and then have problems with getting to sleep the next night. They may get very distressed at the effect this has on their planned activities, e.g. missing the bus for college, yet be unable to sort out their routine alone and without support.

> Sam stayed up late one night to watch a *Star Trek* special. He overslept the next morning and was late for work. He was not sleepy that evening so he watched a late-night movie, and read a book, finally going to bed at 4am. He did not wake up until 2pm the next day and so missed work altogether. By the end of the week Sam was awake all night and sleeping all day. He was then alarmed by a call from his boss saying he was sacked.

Research studies have shown that the sleep patterns of people with AS are different to those of most people. They may find it hard to fit in with other people's sleep routines. Often, their staying up late bothers those they live with because they are noisy, failing to realise they will wake others up. This can cause many problems for people with AS and the people who live with or near them.

MANAGING MONEY

Some people with AS can have major problems with managing their money, despite being able to understand numbers and add up. They often fail to budget. For example they may choose not to spend money on boring things like rent or electricity, but instead choose to spend it on their hobbies or special interests. Because of their social difficulties the person may also be naïve and vulnerable to exploitation. Often the problems only become obvious when things go badly wrong.

> Gary has problems with money. He knows how to add up and can recognise coins and notes, but he doesn't understand how a bank account works and he forgets to pay his bills. One day he lost his rent book for his flat. He didn't know how to get another one, and didn't tell anyone he had lost it. Nobody said anything for a long time, so he thought it was OK, and he spent the money on other things. One day he got a letter from the council threatening to evict him.

Other people with AS may be very resistant to spending their money and may hoard it in the bank. They may go without many things that they need, and may lose friends because of their reluctance to spend money when it is their turn to pay.

✍ *Daily living skills – Trouble-shooting*

Eating

- If eating is a problem, work out a balanced diet made up of the foods that the person with AS enjoys. Put this into a timetable that they can consult, so they know what they will be eating when.

- Plates with sections can be helpful for individuals who do not like foods to touch. They can also be used to promote a balanced diet by explaining that each section must contain one of the three food groups (protein, carbohydrate, vegetable/fruit).

- If the person with AS eats a narrow range of foods it may be worth trying to introduce foods that are as similar as possible to the foods they currently eat. So, if someone likes soft food and does not eat enough vegetables, you could try thick vegetable soup, houmous or guacamole.

- If the person you support is restricting their diet, and is losing a lot of weight, then you should ask them to see their doctor. They may need to see a dietician.

Clothing

- If the person with AS does not like wearing new clothes it may help to put these through the washing with their other clothes a few times, before suggesting that they wear them. This way, they will be softened and will smell the same as their other clothes.

- If wearing the same colour is a habit, then try introducing a similar colour but slightly different from their usual choice. For example, if they like wearing black all the time, see if they will accept navy blue.

- Try to ensure that the clothes they buy are natural materials and soft fabrics, as these are less likely to be irritating to a sensitive skin.

- Discuss the right kinds of clothes for different kinds of weather, or different situations, and see if your client can make the link. However, some people with AS seem not to notice temperature differences.

Personal hygiene and daily routines

Clear written rules and contracts can be very helpful in motivating people with AS to understand why some things are not a good idea, and why other things are expected. Generally they like rules because it makes things clearer for them and more predictable.

- Rooms must be cleaned once a week to keep them hygienic.

- If the person with AS refuses to clean, then negotiate that someone else will be allowed in their room to do basic cleaning.

- No food should be kept in bedrooms because it will attract mice.

Use visual prompts and timetables to improve memory and organisation, and where possible, build structure in. For example, a sorter laundry basket (whites/coloureds/delicates), with each section the size of a machine load, makes washing much easier.

Give clear information on what is healthy and why it needs to be done, and give praise for any small improvements, and for all tasks successfully completed.

Explain the gains that can come from good personal hygiene to the person with AS:

'If you look smart and clean and smell nice people are more likely to want to be your friend. You will feel more comfortable, and your skin will stay healthy.'

Managing money

If the person with AS struggles to manage their money, help them to work out a budget. Creative use of different accounts, direct debits and standing orders can help them control their spending and pay their bills on time. For example: one account for bills and one for spending money.

If the person becomes concerned that you are trying to spend their money, consider an advocate (someone, usually a volunteer in the UK, who will act for the person, to represent them and communicate their wishes). However, this person will have to understand the difficulties of someone with AS. If you are concerned that the AS person is not capable of managing their money, and they dislike you becoming involved, it may be wise to seek legal advice.

7 Managing Emotions

People with Asperger Syndrome (AS) frequently need help to understand and manage their:

- the type and range of emotions experienced
- fight or flight
- angry outbursts.

EMOTIONS EXPERIENCED

People with AS may experience a narrower range of emotions than most people. However, these emotions can be very intense. The most frequent negative emotions experienced by individuals with AS are:

- anxiety
- anger/frustration
- sadness
- loneliness/isolation.

People with AS often have difficulty managing these emotions. Often this is because they have difficulty in identifying their feelings or labelling them. As a result they can have difficulty expressing what they are feeling. They may also have difficulty connecting the emotion with the event that caused it and hence may not be able to explain why they reacted in a particular way.

These difficulties can be experienced even by those who appear to have good verbal skills. It is important to be aware of the different ways that people with AS deal with emotions, to be able to support them in managing their negative feelings.

We have already seen that people with AS find it hard to see things from other people's perspectives. This can complicate their emotional responses, and their responses to other people's emotions.

They may over-react to the behaviour of someone else, because they are upset by it. They assume that it has been done deliberately to upset them, even when it is clear to others that this is not so. For example:

'Peter moved house because he didn't like me and wanted to upset me.'

They often fail to see how their behaviour has provoked someone else:

'The man on the bus shouted at me angrily for no reason.'

(In fact, the person with AS had pushed into the queue without realising that they had done so.)

They may often fail to take responsibility for their own emotional reactions:

'He made me angry, so it is his fault that I hit him.'

Sometimes people with AS can upset other people by expressing inappropriate emotions, such as laughing when someone is hurt. This can make them disliked by those around them, who see them as heartless or as enjoying other people's misfortunes.

Exercise

Try and recall a time in your past when you may have experienced a very strong emotion, which was triggered by what seemed, on the face of it, a minor event.

How did this make you feel?

How did other people react to you?

What would it feel like always to have emotional reactions that were so intense and unexpected?

How might this affect your behaviour, and the way that other people might react to you?

With their permission, observe the person with AS who you are supporting over a few days. Take particular notice of times when you think they are responding emotionally to a situation. Record how you think the person was feeling:

Next time you see the person behaving this way ask them how they feel. What did they say? (*Be careful if you think they are feeling angry.*)

Was the person able to tell you what they felt?

Did the answer match your guess?

FIGHT OR FLIGHT

Anxiety and anger are survival emotions. They make up what is called the 'fight or flight' response. When we are faced with a dangerous situation our bodies prepare to attack the danger (*fight*) or run away (*flight*). The physical sensations of anger and anxiety are the result of the release of hormones causing the heart to pump blood away from the digestive tract and other less important areas of the body, towards the large muscles, in preparation for vigorous activity.

In today's society we need these emotions less than we did when we lived in the jungle, but these responses are part of our biological make-up. Anger or anxiety can be triggered by all kinds of experiences, sometimes when it is impossible to do what we are programmed to do. For example, the boss at work may make us angry, but it is not acceptable to start a fight with them!

Anxiety can make us want to run away when we can't, and this can make us feel very uncomfortable. It is difficult to run away from a situation at work, even if we feel that we would like to.

The physical effects of anger or anxiety can include:

- difficulty concentrating

- difficulty relaxing

- feeling butterflies in the tummy

- trembling or shaking

- tension

- sweating (clammy hands)

- light-headedness

- palpitations

- dizziness

- dry mouth.

Anxiety is usually associated with a feeling of tension, fear or nervousness. People with AS tend to have higher levels of anxiety than the general population, even when nothing unusual seems to be happening to them. Their anxiety can be increased by:

- dealing with changes in the physical and social environment

- routines and rituals being disrupted

- worrying about dealing with social situations

- confusion about other people's reactions

- difficulties solving problems

- difficulty predicting what might happen in any given situation.

As we have already discussed, it may be possible to reduce or remove some of these causes of anxiety by careful management. As people with AS have naturally high levels of anxiety, even when their lives are running smoothly, it is important to build relaxing activities into their daily routine. You may need to find out what works for them by trial and error, as they are unlikely to be able to tell you what they find relaxing.

Exercise

Observe how the person with AS who you support responds to their different daily activities.

Rate each activity as to how relaxed the person is at the start and end of the activity on a scale of:

1 = so tense they are about to explode to 10 = so relaxed they are almost asleep.

Use these headings.

Activity	Score at start of the activity	Score at end

Now look at how much time the person spends doing activities that are exciting or stressful, as against those that appear to be relaxing or routine. Does the person have a good balance of relaxing, exciting and routine activities?

If not, how can you change the balance of activities, so the person you support might become less anxious?

While anxiety is a big problem for people with AS, they can also have problems managing their anger. Their difficulties with social situations may mean that:

- they do not understand a situation

- they are misunderstood, even when acting with the best of intentions

- they misunderstand other people's reactions or behaviour towards them.

In addition, it may happen that the person with AS becomes an easy target for bullies who will tease and push them to their limit, in anticipation of the enjoyment of watching them explode.

People with AS may also have great difficulty managing their stress, leading to a major build-up of tension. Pent-up feelings of anger and frustration can fuel angry outbursts, such as shouting, swearing, aggression to others, or damage to property. Alternatively, they may turn their anger inwards, resulting in self-harm.

ANGRY OUTBURSTS

These angry outbursts may appear to come 'out of the blue', without warning signs, and can be triggered by a simple question or a small demand. This is because the person with AS has built up a high level of frustration over a period of time (this may be hours or days) as the result of many small annoyances, and this last demand is the straw that broke the camel's back.

Once this gets to a certain point the next annoyance, however small, will trigger an angry outburst. This often leads to people with AS being seen as 'unpredictable' or 'unreasonable'. Their behaviour will only make sense if you have been able to see the whole series of annoyances. Sadly, they are unlikely to be able to explain this to you.

It can be very helpful, in understanding such outbursts, to consider the behaviour that triggered it as 'the last straw' rather than the reason for the outburst.

Exercise

Can you recall an occasion when you lost your temper completely over a very small issue?

What triggered the outburst? Was it 'the final straw'?

How did that last demand make you feel?

What events led up to this?

What was the 'real' reason you lost your temper?

Imagine how it would be often to feel as you did just before you lost your temper.

For most people with AS it is likely that there will be subtle signs of their build-up of anger that are easily missed. For example:

- stopping work because they do not know what to do next

- fingers in the ears because the situation is too noisy

- gazing into the distance to block out the situation

- going straight to their room on coming home from work, rather than making a cup of tea.

These warning signs will vary from individual to individual. When you get to know a person with AS well, you will probably be able to spot their warning signs.

There may also be a behavioural hierarchy that indicates increasing distress. For example:

1. relaxed and smiling

2. fidgeting and rearranging personal possessions

3. raised voice

4. increasingly rapid speech

5. hitting furniture/slamming doors

6. shouting and verbal abuse

7. hitting out at other people.

Unfortunately, some people with AS learn very quickly that aggression gets them what they want. If people back off when they shout or lash out, then they will soon learn that this helps them:

- to be left alone

- to watch the TV programme they want

- to eat the food they wish to eat

- to sit in a particular chair

- to keep people out of their room.

Once this method of getting what the person wants is learned, it is very hard to change and may need expert help. Watch for the early signs of this pattern, and try to manage outbursts so that they have a neutral outcome for the person rather than giving them what they want.

However, it is also important to listen and, as far as possible, to respect the person's wishes, so that they are not driven to trying to get what they want by aggression.

Finally, some apparently unprovoked outbursts or aggression can be the result of a grudge. People with AS often have a strong sense of right and wrong, and of what is fair. If someone has upset them, or is perceived to have treated them unfairly, they may hold on to a grudge until they see an opportunity for retaliation.

Jasmin was seen by one of her lecturers to walk up behind a fellow student in the lunch queue. For no apparent reason she hit him very hard on the back of the head and then walked away. When Jasmin was told off for this assault she was very angry. She considered this attack was justified because the other student had pushed her in the bus queue several days ago.

Exercise

Observe the person you support carefully, so that you build up an understanding of the situations that make them angry. Record what was happening immediately before they became angry. Include the time and day, what they were doing, who else was there and what happened afterwards. It is important to note what they did and how everyone responded to them.

Day/time	Behaviour	Situation	Activity	Consequences

Are any patterns apparent?

Can you see any sequence of escalating distress prior to the angry behaviour?

Does the person seem to achieve something they want through getting angry?

Can they achieve that result without getting angry?

See if you can find ways that this might be achieved.

✍ *Managing emotions – Trouble-shooting*

It may help to create a picture dictionary of feelings, with a description of how each one feels. This might help the person with AS to understand their own feelings, and learn how to label them. This, in turn, could help others to understand how the person with AS is feeling.

Managing anxiety

Try new activities that may help the person you support to relax, e.g.

- music

- aromatherapy diffusers

- quiet time alone

- going for a walk

- repetitive tasks such as tidying the sock drawer or doing easy sums

- rhythmic physical activity such as trampolining, yoga or tai chi

- fishing

- jacuzzi, sauna or whirlpool bath

- reflexology, massage or foot spa

- contact with animals, e.g. patting a dog or stroking a cat.

New activities should always be tried for the first time when the person is calm. You may need to try an activity more than once before making a decision. Add any that the person enjoys, and which help them to stay calm, to their schedule of weekly activities.

Physical exercise can be excellent for reducing stress, especially walking, running and swimming. However, do not be tempted to suggest team sports such as football. The social complexities of these games can be extremely stressful for people with AS and this is likely to undo the benefits of the exercise.

Check out how much caffeine the person is drinking. Caffeine is found in tea, coffee, cola drinks, some sports drinks and chocolate. Too much caffeine increases anxiety symptoms. Agree with them to try and reduce their intake or switch to decaffeinated versions.

If the person regularly becomes so anxious that it is difficult to manage, they need to be referred for professional help to manage anxiety. Sometimes people with AS may also need the help of medication. They will need to discuss this with their doctor or a psychiatrist.

Managing anger

Excessive anger can be destructive and dangerous. It is important to develop ways of managing someone whose anger is frequently out of control.

- Brainstorm with others who know the person well, to find things that will help the person to calm down and thus de-escalate difficult situations. Share your knowledge with everyone who cares for them.

- Stay calm when faced with someone who is getting angry. Use a calming voice and non-threatening body language when communicating with them. Keep sentences short and simple.

- If this does not work, you may have to let the outburst happen, then talk about it later when the person has calmed down. Do not try to discuss the problem in detail with them at the time; they won't be able to think rationally when they are very emotionally aroused.

- It is important after an outburst to consider what the warning signs may have been and see what lessons can be learned for the future. Record these.

If angry outbursts persist, you should help the person seek professional help from the doctor. They may need referral to a psychologist or psychiatrist. For some people 'as required' medication can help to manage angry outbursts. Again the doctor should be able to help with this. Do not leave this problem too long; it can be dangerous to others.

Friends and Relationships

This is perhaps one of the most difficult areas for people with Asperger syndrome (AS). The difficulties they have with social situations in general become magnified when they are trying to establish close relationships:

- friendships and relationships can be confusing

- desire for friendship

- overestimation of abilities

- exploitation

- bullying, teasing and being left out

- impact on self-esteem

- social withdrawal and depression

- social phobias and anxiety.

FRIENDSHIPS AND RELATIONSHIPS CAN BE CONFUSING

Relationships and friendships can be confusing for many people. Personal relationships contain lots of potential for misunderstanding and conflict. The key to successful relationships is often good communication, and we already know that this is something that people with AS struggle with.

If friendships and relationships are difficult for people who have good social skills, imagine how difficult friendships or relationships must be for people with AS. They are likely to experience frequent failure in their attempts to make friends. They have problems with communicating with others, and often don't understand the rules that operate in many social situations. In close relationships these rules can be even more subtle, and they fail without knowing why.

DESIRE FOR FRIENDSHIP

People with AS usually want to make friends with others. Unfortunately, they usually have little idea about how to do this. Often they misread a situation, and think they have a friend when they have not.

> Patrick goes to the Post Office to get his benefits. He likes to go because he thinks the people behind the counter are his friends. He spends ages talking to whoever serves him, not noticing their discomfort and the annoyance of the queue behind him.

It is clear that Patrick has no understanding of what a friend really is; this is very common in people with AS. Often they think that anyone who talks to them is a friend. This is particularly true of less able people with AS. People who support those with AS need to be aware of this, and to discreetly check the nature of so called friendships. People with AS are vulnerable and are often exploited because of this need to have friends.

More able people with AS have usually realised quite early in life that they can't make friends like other people do. Often they can become quite depressed about this.

When people with AS do try to make friends or begin relationships, their unusual behaviour can often put people off, and they may withdraw quickly. Repeated experiences like this may lead the person to give up trying to make friends. However, this does not mean that they do not want relationships with others. Unfortunately, even when they succeed in forming a relationship with someone, it may go disastrously wrong. Sometimes the other person will struggle on for years, making allowances and trying to make the relationship work. Usually they get to a point where they give up, leaving the person with AS confused and hurt.

OVERESTIMATION OF ABILITIES

Even the most able people with AS struggle with close relationships. Because they appear very able in some ways, their behaviour may appear to be very deliberately rude. People do not understand their difficulties. In other cases the person may just seem odd or very eccentric to others.

Adam is a very able young man with a passion for football. He can tell you the dates of many past football events and who was playing. When he goes to the pub to watch the football he cannot understand why the other supporters do not want to be his friends. In fact, the others avoid him because he insists on talking over the match commentary. In addition, he interrupts other people's conversations and they get very annoyed with him. Adam gets very upset that he has no friends, and cannot understand why the others avoid or ignore him when he goes to the pub.

People with AS are often misunderstood. Because they talk fluently and have a good long-term memory, they are expected also to have good social understanding and skills. They often alienate others without knowing why. Sadly, this can still happen even when they are trying hard to do things right.

EXPLOITATION

In some cases, people with AS are so desperate to make friends that they are taken advantage of by others. They will often naïvely accept being exploited by others in order to keep the 'friendship' going. They may lend others money which is not paid back, or end up doing other people's chores for them.

> Jeremy thought he had lots of friends at his local pub. People were always very pleased to see him, and would exchange greetings with him. He would buy them drinks and did not seem to mind that they never bought drinks for him. However, once his money was spent, the people soon drifted off and Jeremy would go home alone.

Exploitation is also discussed in the chapter about sexuality and relationships.

BULLYING, TEASING AND BEING LEFT OUT

Behaviour that is thought of as odd by others can result in teasing and bullying. If the person with AS is thought to be rude they may find themselves left out of social activities by others. As you would expect, this can be very distressing for the person with AS. They will not understand why others do not like them, let alone why they are excluded and in some cases bullied and teased. Unfortunately, people with AS often make easy targets for bullies as they are easily provoked, and bullies will enjoy seeing them explode, and possibly get into trouble as a result.

IMPACT ON SELF-ESTEEM

Repeated social failure and being victimised by bullies can have a huge impact on someone's self-esteem. Not surprisingly, people with

AS are often found to have low self-esteem. Eventually they may give up trying, and withdraw completely.

SOCIAL WITHDRAWAL AND DEPRESSION

This social withdrawal and low self-esteem can lead to depression. The individual may experience extreme feelings of sadness and guilt related to their struggles to form friendships and relationships with others. They feel a failure and their experiences repeatedly confirm these feelings. This can put them at risk of suicide in extreme cases.

SOCIAL PHOBIAS AND ANXIETY

We have seen that high levels of anxiety are common in people with AS. Repeated failure in social situations can only make this worse. In some cases, this heightened anxiety may result in the person trying to escape from or avoid social situations altogether, and can develop into a significant social phobia (fear of social situations) or into agoraphobia (fear of leaving home). If this happens, they may need professional help.

Exercise

From your own knowledge of the person you support, draw a plan of their social circle. Draw a stick figure at the centre of a series of concentric circles. The inner circle is for intimate relationships, the next circle is for family and friends, the next for acquaintances and the final one for people they come into contact with regularly, such as the doctor, but who are not friends.

Does this person have a rich social network?

Next, ask the person you support to complete their version of the assessment with you.

Is it the same as your version? If the person has added people you had not identified, or has put them in a more intimate circle than you would expect, you may want to talk about what friends are, and why they see them as a friend. However, be careful of destroying their illusions. Provided that there is no exploitation involved, it may help them to believe that they have friendships, even if they are not what we would understand by the term. You may need to work on helping them develop real new friends instead.

Are there big gaps, or empty circles? Check with the person how they feel about this. It is important to do this in a neutral way, as you do not want to make them anxious about a lack of friends if they are happy with their current network. (Bear in mind that people with AS often have lower expectations of what a friend will be. They are often happy with quite superficial contacts.)

If they would like help to make new friends, then work through the following questions with them:

- What do they have to offer friends? (What are their good points?)

- What might be getting in the way of them making friends?

You may need to use specific prompts, e.g.:

- appearance (clothes, hair, cleanliness)

- body language (eye contact, posture)

- starting a conversation

- the things they talk about

- the way they behave.

- Do they go to the right places to meet new people? Make a plan with the person using ideas from the trouble-shooting section to help them find, make and keep new friends.

✍ Friends and relationships – Trouble-shooting

General tips

Accept that the social needs of individuals with AS are different. Many people may like to have plenty of time alone and need less social contact. They are often happy just to exchange a few friendly words with people.

Offer sympathy and support to those who are bullied or teased by others and teach them how to be more assertive. If necessary, take the issue up with school, college or place of work. (You may wish to consult with your line manager/supervisor about how best to approach this.)

If the bullying is happening at home, you could try and teach others sharing this setting with the person about their needs and problems.

Does the person with AS seem confused about what friends really are? If so, help them to understand how friends should and should not behave. Social Stories™ may be helpful in doing this.

Explore with the person what characteristics are desirable in a friend, e.g. fun to be with, loyal, trustworthy, kind, considerate, understanding, etc.

Explore with the person what characteristics are undesirable in a friend, e.g. being disloyal, untrustworthy, cruel, inconsiderate, not understanding, etc.

Discuss with the person who they consider their friends to be (if any) and why they like these people.

Describe and explore with the person the social rules that lead to making friends, e.g. sharing interests, taking turns, helping each other, etc.

Make a visual record of this, perhaps using pictures and symbols, so that it may be reviewed as often as needed.

Making friends

Identify with the person you support practical ways of making friends with new people. It may be helpful to develop these around specific settings where the person already goes, or those that you have identified as places to go to meet potential friends.

For example if attending an evening class, you might suggest that they chat to other people in the class before it starts. They could then ask someone that they like if they would like a coffee in the break. During the break they might talk a bit about the class and maybe ask a few questions about the other person.

It will be important to explain that friendships develop over time and that most people are put off if you try to push things too quickly, or say things such as 'Will you be my friend?'

Help the individual to realise that they may dominate a conversation with their special interest, and try to teach them a range of topics to talk about instead, such as the weather, what they watched on TV last night, the football scores or something similar. Use role-play to practise the ideas you have talked about.

Help them to build basic skills that allow them to maintain friendships, such as how to arrange meetings using the telephone.

Encourage them to seek friends with similar interests.

Help them to build up a network of activities or clubs where others share their interests. Odd social behaviours are sometimes less intrusive if everyone is taking part in the same activity.

Make sure they know how to keep safe. Teach youngsters about 'stranger danger'. Make those of all ages aware of the risks of answering date advertisements, etc. It may be helpful to put down on paper a set of rules for keeping safe.

Be creative. Help the person you support to use alternative ways of communicating, such as internet chat rooms for people with common interests, bearing in mind the need to stay safe, as above.

If, despite all your efforts, the person with AS is still failing to make friends, it may be worth considering whether a professional 'friend', such as a volunteer, or an advocate may be a possibility.

Sexuality and Relationships

For young men with Asperger syndrome (AS) in particular, this is often the area of life which causes them the greatest problems:

- getting started

- first impressions matter

- lack of a sexual relationship

- when people with AS have relationships

- people with AS can be vulnerable

- stalking.

As most of us reach adolescence, we become aware of other people that we find sexually attractive. These attractions can lead first to relationships, and then to sexual contact, if the feelings are mutual. Although people with AS have problems with social situations and meeting people, they often still want to have close relationships and sexual contact with others. As with the rest of us, some people will want heterosexual relationships and some will want homosexual relationships. Do not make assumptions about this.

GETTING STARTED

People with AS often fail to realise when others find them attractive, and struggle to let others know that they find them attractive in an appropriate way.

Exercise

How do you know that someone is interested in you?

What do they say?

What do they do?

Ask friends or colleagues how they let someone know that they fancy them. What do they do, or say?

How did they learn these techniques?

Would the person you support recognise signals of interest such as these?

Would they be able to use these techniques themselves?

A lot of people with AS have low self-esteem as a result of the difficulties that they have experienced. They know that they are different, and so they may not feel confident enough to approach new people, whether to make friends or let them know that they find them attractive. Even if they can pluck up the courage to make an approach, they usually do not know how to show their interest in the right way. Often they can get it very wrong.

Matthew wants a girlfriend. He is desperate to meet someone, so he decides to try and find a girlfriend at the supermarket. He thinks that as there are lots of women of all ages in the supermarket he is sure to find someone there. One day he sees just the girl he fancies and follows her home. He can't understand why she gets angry and threatens to call the police.

The person with AS is unlikely to have any idea why they got it wrong, and can often feel very hurt. Without guidance or support they are likely to get it wrong again, and keep getting it wrong. This constant experience of failure can lead them to give up on a romantic or sexual life altogether in some cases. Sadly, the lack of success does not mean that the interest goes away.

FIRST IMPRESSIONS MATTER

When trying to strike up a new relationship, physical appearance and dress sense can be important. People can be put off by poor appearance, at least initially. However, despite often having a handsome face, or pretty features, people with AS may:

- lack facial expression when they are talking

- not make eye contact with others

- have a strange posture; they may stand slightly stooped or hunched

- have a tendency to move clumsily

- have an unusual choice of clothing or hairstyle

- neglect personal hygiene.

These characteristics are all things that can affect first impressions. Unusual non-verbal behaviour can immediately put someone off, and lead them to decide very early on that this person is not someone that they would find attractive. This is something else that may put people with AS at a disadvantage when it comes to meeting and making a good impression on people that they find attractive. When combined with the problems of coping with social rules and conversation, it is hardly surprising that the person with AS never gets started.

LACK OF A SEXUAL RELATIONSHIP

This total failure to establish a satisfactory relationship will often lead to severe sexual frustration. To relieve this the person may resort to masturbation. This need not be a problem. It is a normal process, but the person with AS may not always approach this in a socially acceptable way.

It is important to accept that the person may wish to use masturbation to release sexual tension, but there should be clear rules about where this is acceptable. You may also need to think through how the staff team will cope if the person wishes to access pornography.

WHEN PEOPLE WITH AS HAVE RELATIONSHIPS

Occasionally, however, people with AS are lucky in love. They find someone that they like and enjoy spending time with. Unfortunately, the person's success at this stage is often short-lived.

It sometimes happens that a young person with AS is physically attractive and on the basis of that alone will attract a series of partners. Usually these relationships do not last, once the partner realises what the person is really like, and sees their odd behaviour.

Occasionally, though, some people with AS will marry and have a family. The partner may struggle on for years to make the relationship work, especially where there are children. Sadly, though, they often get to a point of being completely demoralised and give up, sometimes after many years. This can provoke a crisis which brings the person with AS to mental health services, often depressed, bewildered and hurt.

Eddie has been married for a number of years. He is a good looking man, and easily attracted his wife, although she was puzzled about how reserved he seemed. Over the years they have been together she has become more and more hurt and puzzled by his behaviour. He never remembers birthdays or anniversaries and can't understand why this upsets her. However, he never forgets a football match, and travels to all the away games. He still does this even when the game clashes with an important family event. Eddie does not tell his wife that he loves her, because he assumes she knows. He often treats her, she feels, as part of the furniture. Yet when she tells him one day that she is leaving, Eddie is devastated. He really cannot understand what he has done wrong.

The most successful relationships for people with AS seem to be when they get together. There have been quite a number of occasions when people have made successful marriages with another person who has AS, or sometimes adult autism. These relationships seem to work for the same reasons that most relationships do: the partners understand each other, and share similar views and expectations.

Exercise

Think of a relationship you have had that made you feel valued and loved.

What did the other person do to make you feel that way? (Think about body language, touch, tone of voice, little things they might have done, what they said and when they said it.)

Think of a relationship that made you feel unloved or taken for granted.

What did the person do to make you feel that way? (Think again about body language, touch, tone of voice, things they might have done or not done, what they said and when they said it.)

- Did you ever try to explain how their behaviour made you feel?

- Why do you think the person behaved that way?

- Did you ever ask?

Consider how subtle many of these behaviours are and how often we don't discuss them.

The following issues can also cause problems in relationships. Often there are unspoken expectations about how these things should be shared or dealt with. Consider these issues: what behaviour/actions/responses are OK and not OK in relationships?

Exercise

Issue	OK behaviours	Not OK behaviours
Money matters		
Travelling to see each other		
Chores		
Arguments		
Spending time with other people/hobbies		
Spending time together		

PEOPLE WITH AS CAN BE VULNERABLE

In some cases people with AS want romantic or sexual relationships with others to such a degree that they become involved with people that are totally unsuitable for them.

They may choose people who appear to be a very odd match for them, or they become involved with undesirable people. In these cases, because the person with AS may be getting some of what they want, they may ignore the negative aspects of the relationship. They are content just to have a boy or girlfriend like everyone else. This leaves people with AS very vulnerable to being exploited. People may be abused financially, physically, mentally or sexually.

> Katrina formed a new relationship with Steve. He quickly moved into her flat. She was over the moon that she at last had found a real relationship. However, a few months later, she was distressed to find out her bank account was empty. She mentioned this to Steve. The next morning he had vanished, as had her TV, CD, DVD player and her money for emergencies. Katrina still hopes that Steve will return and cannot see that he was only after a free roof over his head.

This not only affects the person with AS, but can also cause distress for the person's family and carers. Problems like this can put a major strain on the relationship between the person with AS and the people who support them. They may only want the best for them, but their criticisms or advice will not usually be welcome.

Some people with AS also make themselves very vulnerable by behaving in unacceptable ways. They have sexual needs and desires just like everyone else, but for some people with AS these needs are stronger than for others.

People with AS cannot balance their needs and feelings against those of other people. They put their needs and feelings first every time and find it very difficult to understand why anyone else would want something different from what they want.

Unfortunately, not realising that others have their own wishes, thoughts and feelings can result in the person with AS behaving in ways that are offensive or frightening to others.

> Matt realises that most men his age have girlfriends and are beginning to have sex. Matt has a strong desire to be like his peers and has a very high sex drive. He has no idea how to approach girls to show his interest or attraction to them in a socially acceptable way. Matt approached a young girl who was a stranger to him in the street. He grabbed her and tried to touch her breasts and kiss her. Matt had no understanding that he had done anything wrong and when he got in trouble with the police he calmly explained that he was just trying to show her he fancied her and make her his girlfriend.

Fortunately, this is an extreme example, and such behaviour is not common with people with AS. However, it is important to be aware of what can go wrong. Be ready to spot warning signs and take action before something serious occurs. If someone commits an 'offence' of this kind, however innocent the motivation, it can cause great distress to the victim, the person with AS and his carers or family. It can also lead to severe restrictions being placed on the person's freedom.

STALKING

People with AS have a tendency to develop obsessive interests. However, this not only happens in relation to subjects such as trains or TV transmitters, but also can happen towards certain people. Usually this is relatively harmless, although it can be unnerving for the person who is the focus of that interest. More rarely it can develop into stalking.

> When Laura began working at a local supermarket part time, her supervisor was informed of her diagnosis of AS,

and he offered Laura extra support with her work. He gave her his personal phone number so that she could call him if she ever needed any help, or was concerned about her work. Laura misunderstood this attention and thought that he was interested in spending extra time with her as his girlfriend. She began following him and calling his phone regularly, although not just in relation to work. When she did call, Laura often became confused about what to say and just sat listening to her supervisor's voice. She followed him home on numerous occasions. Eventually, Laura was sacked, although her behaviour continued. Consequently, her supervisor felt he had no choice but to involve the police. Laura was very hurt and distressed by this reaction. She couldn't understand why he would want to stop their relationship. She became very obsessed about it, and eventually ill and depressed.

Whilst stalking is rare, it is important when working with people with AS to think carefully about your relationship with them, to minimise the risk of triggering such an obsession.

Exercise

Think about the way you interact with the person with AS that you support. How might they misunderstand your motivation?

Consider the following:

What you might do	Your motivation	Message you may be giving
Giving a birthday card		
Shaking hands		
Hugging them		
Taking them to the cinema		
Taking them to your home		
Telling them you don't have a partner		
Saying where you live		
Touching them when they are distressed		
Letting them hug or kiss you		
Paying a compliment		
Calling them 'Dear' or 'Love'		

Which of these would you advise paid carers not to do?

Having thought about this, are there any things that you do now that you think you should change?

✍ Sexuality and relationships – Trouble-shooting

Getting started

Explore with the person with AS what they are looking for in a relationship and who they find attractive.

If the person's expectations are unrealistic or inappropriate, explore this with them and discuss alternative ways of thinking about relationships.

Use Social Stories™ and role-play to build their confidence to approach appropriate people that they find attractive.

Find out about the places they visit regularly. Is it likely they will find what they are looking for there? If these places are not suitable, think of alternative places the person could go in order to meet someone with similar interests:

- clubs (think about different types of clubs)

- activities

- classes

- hobbies.

Bearing in mind their difficulties and vulnerabilities, think carefully about the type of people likely to be there (or check the place out first). Try to choose groups and places where the person will fit in best, and feel most comfortable.

Speed dating can be very appealing for people with AS as they do not have to think of too much to say, and they have a means of getting away if they do not like someone. The issue of vulnerability will still have to be considered though.

Actively organise social events and invite suitable people (but don't be too narrow minded about who is suitable!). You may find useful contacts through the National Autistic Society website, who also help those with AS.

Be cautious about suggesting pubs or bars as a way of meeting people. Even if someone does not have a problem with alcohol at present, this may develop if they spend a lot of time alone in bars.

They may also meet the wrong kind of people and be vulnerable in such a place.

Consider using dating agencies. If the person is of limited ability, there are now some specialist agencies for people who also have a learning disability.

First impressions

Explain to the person the impact that first impressions of physical appearance can have on relationships:

> 'It is not nice to wear dirty or smelly clothes when going out to meet someone.'

Use Social Stories™ to emphasise the importance of being well presented.

Explore whether the person with AS would themselves be put off by someone looking dirty or untidy.

It may help to build the person's confidence by telling them their good features. Give them praise when they have made an effort with their appearance. However, think carefully how you phrase this, as you do not want to create the impression that you fancy them:

> 'The women at the club will think you look smart,'

is much safer than

> 'Wow, you look hot in that!'

Having a relationship

Discuss with the person with AS what is and is not OK in a relationship. Find out what they think is acceptable or desirable and what is not.

It may help to use Social Stories™ and role-play (be careful with role-play that they understand that you are acting and do not mistake this for a real situation). It may help to do this with a group of people with similar problems, if possible.

Encourage the individual to be open, and discuss any worries or concerns they have about relationships. However, this needs to be with someone that they know and trust.

Being vulnerable

It is important for someone with AS to have some understanding of what is and is not OK in close relationships, as discussed above. Once this is clear, they may be a little more aware if others are exploiting them.

Explore 'give and take' in relationships with the person with AS.

Use Social Stories™ to discuss imaginary relationships where someone is being mistreated. Ask the person with AS what they would do. If you feel that the person's response is likely to leave them vulnerable to exploitation, discuss suitable alternatives with them.

Note down these discussions and make them into a book about keeping safe in relationships, so that they can refer to it in future.

Think about your own vulnerability and be aware of how your actions could be misunderstood by the person that you support.

Think about how you can meet the need to be warm and friendly with the person you support, without risking misinterpretation.

Safer examples of being friendly:

- If they visit your home, include another client and another member of staff in the party.

- Give them a present and card for their birthday from 'the staff team' or 'everyone at the home' rather than from you personally.

- Put things in simple words rather than using physical contact, e.g. 'I'm sorry you are upset', rather than giving the person a hug.

- Be explicit about your motivations, e.g. 'Yes, I like you but I am here because it is my job.'

If the person with AS who you support has major and enduring problems relating to sex or relationships, it is advisable to help the person to seek professional help. Talk to their doctor first.

10 Mental Health

Because of all their other difficulties, people with Asperger syndrome (AS) are particularly prone to developing mental health problems:

- depression
- social phobia
- self-harm and suicidal ideas or attempts
- obsessive compulsive disorder.

However, AS itself is not a mental health problem and people with AS do not *always* develop mental health problems.

The following difficulties may lead to the development of mental health problems for some:

- feeling unable to cope with mainstream education
- having limited access to further education and support
- having repeated difficulties with getting and keeping a job
- having a very limited circle of friends, and little social support, if any
- having difficult family relations

- perceiving themselves as a social failure

- being unable to cope with everyday, simple problems.

Most of us have a network of friends and family that we can turn to when we face problems. People with AS may not have these supports, or they may simply not think to ask for help. They often feel very isolated.

In addition, they are often acutely aware that they are different from others, even though they do not understand why they fail. This awareness becomes painfully apparent during teenage years and young adulthood. This is a time when we learn how to cope in most social situations, including making friends, forming relationships and dealing with strangers. It is important to be aware of the symptoms of mental health problems that may begin to develop when a person fails to cope.

DEPRESSION

Depression is extremely common in young people with AS, but can occur at any age. The following behaviours can be symptoms of depression:

- prolonged sadness or crying

- withdrawal

- loss of appetite, or excessive comfort eating

- regular difficulty with sleeping, waking up very early or oversleeping

- extreme agitation, anxiety or restlessness

- low self-esteem, especially self-loathing/feelings of guilt/ worthlessness

- loss of pleasure in previously pleasurable activities.

To decide if someone is seriously depressed it is very important to understand what is usual for that person. For example, it is normal for many people with AS to spend a lot of time alone. However, for someone who is usually fairly sociable, this may be a symptom of depression.

Behaviour	Usual personality	Asperger syndrome	Depression?
Sadness/ crying	Aaron misses living with his family; he feels sad when he thinks about this. When his family leave Aaron cries and seeks comfort from members of staff.	Aaron feels sad that he is different to other teenagers; he can't understand why he doesn't have any friends. Aaron tells staff that this makes him feel sad and angry inside.	Recently Aaron has been extremely tearful and cries for no obvious reason. His mood is constantly low.
Withdrawal	Aaron is bubbly and friendly. Despite struggling with social occasions he enjoys spending time with people he knows well on a one to one basis.	Aaron dislikes being in groups of people that he doesn't know; he finds it intimidating. When this is the case Aaron will go to his bedroom.	Aaron has spent the majority of the last week in bed sleeping. He refuses to spend time with any of the staff on a one to one basis and insists that he be left alone.
Appetite	Aaron really enjoys his food and has a sweet tooth.	Aaron is very restricted as to what foods he will eat; he dislikes any food with red sauce.	Aaron is over-eating; he has been hoarding chocolate in his room and binge eating. When staff ask him about this, Aaron becomes very defensive and tearful.

Behaviour	Usual personality	Asperger syndrome	Depression?
Anxiety levels	Aaron is generally quite an anxious person.	Aaron needs a lot of reassurance about seeing his family. He may repeatedly ask staff about when they are next visiting.	Aaron's concerns about when he will next see his family have become very intense. Despite having been given a diary with visits outlined on it, Aaron repeats the date and time of the next visit to himself over and over again.
Low self-esteem	Aaron is not a very confident person and lacks self-esteem.	Aaron particularly lacks confidence when meeting new people.	Aaron has recently expressed feeling worthless and says that no one would notice if he wasn't here any more.
Loss of pleasure	Aaron usually likes to keep very active and enjoys playing sport, especially cricket. He likes to go to watch the local cricket match every Sunday.	Aaron watches videos of cricket over and over again. He can tell you the names of every member of the England squad and their dates of birth.	Aaron has not been to a cricket match for three weeks. He prefers to lie in bed and watch videos of cricket instead.

Exercise

Monitor the person you support for two weeks. Is there anything they are doing or not doing that makes you feel they may be depressed?

Think about the example above, and relate the symptoms of depression so far described to what you have observed.

- What part of the behaviour is characteristic of the person's normal personality?

- What part of the behaviour is characteristic of AS?

- What part of the behaviour is unusual for the person and possibly related to depression?

Put your findings into a table:

Behaviour	Personality	Asperger syndrome	Depression?
Sadness/crying			
Withdrawal			
Appetite			
Anxiety levels			
Low self-esteem			
Loss of pleasure			

If you notice five or more of these symptoms, it is possible that the individual you are caring for is clinically depressed.

If this is the case, it is important that you ask for specialist help and support. You may do this via his doctor, who may refer to the local community mental health team, psychology services or psychiatry services, so that the person receives the support that they need.

SOCIAL PHOBIA

Many people with AS become anxious about social situations because of their repeated experiences of failure. If this fear develops to the point where they are afraid to go out, or meet anyone new, then they may need professional help. A true social phobia is a disorder whereby the person experiences unreasonable and overwhelming fear and anxiety related to social situations:

- They may fear humiliation or embarrassment in front of others.

- They may fear others looking at them or criticising them.

- They may fear meeting new people.

When severe, these anxieties can provoke panic attacks, whereby the person may experience the following:

- difficulty breathing, with a strong, fast heartbeat

- paralysing feelings of terror

- sweating, trembling, shaking, dizziness

- chest pains and/or feelings of choking

- unavoidable thoughts of death, and fear that they are dying.

Unfortunately, once a person has had a panic attack in a particular situation, they are likely to do everything they can to avoid this situation in the future. The fear of further panic attacks increases the chance of one happening again, so a vicious circle develops. Eventually they may end up avoiding going out at all.

If you suspect that the person you are working with may have developed a social phobia, it is important to refer them on for specialist help. Once again, this may be done via the doctor.

SELF-HARM AND SUICIDAL IDEAS OR ATTEMPTS

People with serious mental health problems are more likely to inflict harm upon themselves than on other people. People with AS are also at a higher risk of self-harm or suicide than the general population. For example, in one study, out of 22 males with AS, 5 had attempted suicide by early adulthood (Wing 1981).

Risk signs

The most obvious sign is a direct statement from the person expressing a wish to self harm, or commit suicide or otherwise die. It should also raise concern if there is direct or indirect evidence of them thinking about or planning to harm themselves. While not everyone who threatens self-harm or suicide goes on to do it, this is not a risk to take. Refer the person immediately to a mental health team. The team will make an assessment considering:

- the level of risk the person poses to themselves

- whether they can give reassurance about safety

- circumstances that are likely to make things worse

- how help can be made available at any time.

If you are working with someone with AS who you suspect is at risk of self-harm or suicide, contact their doctor as soon as possible to ensure that they are provided with maximum support. If this cannot be arranged quickly enough, or there is a crisis out of hours, it may be better to take them to Accident and Emergency at your local hospital where they can be assessed by the duty psychiatrist. The psychiatrist will be able to recommend admission to a mental health ward if this is necessary.

OBSESSIVE COMPULSIVE DISORDER

Obsessive compulsive disorder (OCD) is an anxiety disorder characterised by troubling repetitive thoughts, feelings and behaviour. Because people with AS tend to be anxious, and to develop rituals and fixed routines, they are often wrongly diagnosed with this condition.

However, like anyone else, it is possible that someone with AS may also develop OCD. The difference is usually that, in their normal state of mind, the rituals and routines are comforting and make them feel safe. In OCD these begin to take control of the person, and they will endlessly check and repeat their behaviour without being comforted by it. Indeed the behaviour is driven by extreme fear that something terrible will happen otherwise.

Obsessions

These are thoughts that run through the person's mind over and over again. These can be frightening or upsetting and the person feels that they have no control over them. They are usually ideas about harm coming to the person themselves or to those they care about.

Compulsions

These are strong, almost irresistible, urges to carry out a particular action or set of actions. Usually these activities are driven by a fear that some catastrophe will happen if the person doesn't carry them out. These can be activities such as:

- hand washing
- ordering
- checking
- counting
- repeating words.

The compulsions feel out of control. The person will feel increasing anxiety as the urge to carry out the action builds up. They will then feel forced to carry out the behaviour, almost against their will. Once the behaviour is completed they may feel a brief period of calm and relaxation before the urge starts to build up again. This may spiral out of control until the person spends much of their time carrying out compulsive acts. In contrast to the person with AS who is contentedly working through their usual routines, the person with OCD will often remain highly agitated as they carry out their compulsions. Thus, a diagnosis of OCD should only be given to someone with AS if their rituals appear out of control and no longer give them comfort. McDougle and colleagues (1995) carried out a study which confirmed these differences. They found the following types of obsessions and behaviour:

Asperger syndrome	Obsessive compulsive disorder
Repetitive ordering	Compelling
Hoarding	Often related to anxieties about
Telling or asking	contamination, e.g. fear of germs
Touching or tapping	Sexual
Self-harming or mutilating (if this occurs seek professional help)	Religious
	Somatic (bodily feelings)
	Avoiding disaster

Compare these individuals:

Albert has a huge collection of stamps. Every day he spends hours looking through his collection. He goes through the albums over and over again, showing them to anyone who is nearby and will listen. His support worker is frustrated as Albert neglects his household chores in order to do this. However, when the support worker checks on Albert, he smiles and offers to show her his collection. Albert does not mind leaving his stamps to attend his church group, or to go to watch Western films, which he also loves.

Walter can't stand having lights on at night. He insists that his family sit in darkness every evening. This includes not having any light from the television. Instead of going to his room, he sits in the family room to check that his family do not watch TV or switch any lights on. This causes Walter's family a lot of stress. If they do attempt to switch on the lights or television, he becomes very aggressive and sometimes violent towards them. Walter isn't able to control his behaviour and becomes very upset and apologetic after his outbursts. He does not understand why his family cannot just live without the lights on.

Andy had a compulsion to shower, and this was so strong that he would spend all night in the shower, using huge amounts of hot water and not getting any sleep. When he finally got to bed he was exhausted. He would then sleep all day, get up in the evening and start showering again. He became violent if anyone tried to get him out of the shower. When asked why he showered he was not sure, but he said that he could not stop, as he was convinced that something bad would happen to him.

Albert clearly does not have OCD. He has a slightly annoying ritual that gives him great pleasure. This is typical of AS.

Walter's compulsion is less common, but still not unusual in people with AS, who feel they need to control others to feel safe. His distress seems related to others not co-operating with his compulsion rather than the behaviour itself. Would it be a problem if he lived on his own?

Andy is not able to explain his behaviour, but it has become a serious problem for him, in that it has taken over his life. He is dogged by the fear that something awful will happen if he does not stay in the shower, but there is little sense that this is something which is a positive choice. He feels driven to do it by his fear. This is characteristic of OCD.

Note down the rituals and repetitive behaviour shown by the person that you support. Include details of where and when they occur, and how anxious they were before, during and after the behaviour.

Do they appear distressed by the behaviour?

Ask them about these behaviours. Can they explain why they do them?

If they appear relaxed and say they enjoy the behaviour, it is unlikely to be a compulsion, however annoying its impact on other people. However, if they wish to stop but can't, it may well be a compulsion and a symptom of OCD.

If you suspect they may have OCD, once again you should seek professional help. Both psychological treatments and drugs may help.

✍ Mental Health – Trouble-shooting

Mental health problems need professional help. There is little that you can do beyond being generally supportive and helpful. However, your emotional and practical support can make a huge difference in helping the person to follow the advice and treatment recommendations of their mental health professionals.

If you think that the person that you are working with is suffering from any of the mental health problems that have been discussed in this section, it is advisable that you refer them for professional help. Ideally this should be with their consent. However, if there is a risk to the person or to other people you should seek help even if the person does not wish you to.

Contact the person's doctor, who will discuss possible referrals to the following services:

- Primary Care Mental Health Team (PCMHT) or Community Team for People with Learning Disabilities (CTPLD), depending on their level of ability.

- Psychiatry

- Psychology

- Occupational Therapy

- Psychotherapy.

It is important to be aware of whether or not the person you support has a learning disability, as this makes a difference as to which services they can access. The CTPLD will be able to help with a wider range of issues.

PCMHT will only be able to offer help with serious mental health problems and may have less expertise in working with people with AS. In some areas there will be one or two people with specialist knowledge who may be able to help, but resources in the UK are usually very limited.

References

Gillberg, I.C. and Gilliberg, C. (1989) 'Asperger Syndrome: Some epidemiological Considerations.' A research note. *Journal of Child Psychology and Psychiatry, 30*, 631–638.

Wing, L. (1981) 'Asperger's syndrome: a clinical account'. *Psychological Medicine, 11*, 115–129.

McDougle, C.J., Kresh, L.E., Goodman, W.K., Naylor, S.T., Volkmar, F.R., and Price, L.H. (1995) 'A case-controlled study of repetitive thoughts and behaviour in adults with autistic disorder and obsessive compulsive disorder'. *American Journal of Psychiatry 152(5)*, 772–777.

Additional Reading and Information

Attwood, T. (1998) *Asperger's Syndrome: A Guide for Parents and Professionals.* London: Jessica Kingsley Publishers.

Attwood, T. (2008) *The Complete Guide to Asperger's Syndrome.* London: Jessica Kingsley Publishers.

Crissey, P. (2004) *Personal Hygiene? What's That Got to Do with Me?* London: Jessica Kingsley Publishers.

Gray, C. (1995) *The New Social Stories Book: Illustrated Edition.* Arlington: Future Horizons.

Hodgdon, L.A. (1995) *Visual Strategies for Improving Communication: Practical Supports for School and Home.* Troy, Michigan: Quirk Roberts Publishing.

Jackson, L. (2002) *Freaks, Geeks and Asperger Syndrome: A User Guide to Adolescence.* London: Jessica Kingsley Publishers.

Smith Myles, B. & Southwick, J. (1999) *Asperger Syndrome and Difficult Moments. Practical Solutions for Tantrums, Rage and Meltdown.* Kansas: Autism & Asperger Publishing Co.

Smith Myles, B., Tapscott Cook, B., Miller, N.E., Rinner, L. and Robbins, L.A. (2001) *Asperger Syndrome and Sensory Issues: Practical Solutions for Making Sense of the World.* London: Jessica Kingsley Publishers.

Willey, L.H. (1999) *Pretending to be Normal: Living with Asperger's Syndrome.* London: Jessica Kingsley Publishers.

Social Stories
Social Stories™ 10.0 (PDF download)

thegreycenter.org – follow the links for Social Stories™. A PDF guide on writing social stories can be purchased from this website. There is also information on courses and publications by Carol Gray.

Index

abilities 28
accents 41
    see also echolalia
advocates 100
agoraphobia *see* social phobia
anger 104, 106
    negative reinforcement 108
    trouble-shooting 110–12
    warning signs 107
anxiety 64, 104
    social phobia 117
    trouble-shooting 110–11
    see also special interest; 'fight or flight' response;
    Obsessive compulsive disorder
awareness of others 67

basic rules of conversation 30
body language 31
budgeting *see* daily living
bullying 116, 119

care plans 11
change 63
    problems with 64

to environment 65, 75
    see also routine
clothes *see* daily living
communication
    trouble-shooting 45–50
communication difficulties 25
    topic changes 29
communication skills 26
Community Team for People with Learning
Disabilities (CTPLD) 147
compulsions 72, 144–6
    see also Obsessive compulsive disorder
concept questions 48
consent 13
consistency 64
control 76
control over others 10
conversation
    ending 31
    maintaining 27
    scripted 27–8
    starting 45
    taking over the 29, 30
    topic changes 28
'conversational tennis' 46